BLUEPRINTS
Pocket Gastroenterology

Blueprints for your pocket!

In an effort to answer a need for high yield review books for the elective rotations, Lippincott Williams & Wilkins now brings you **Blueprints** in pocket size.

These new **Blueprints Pockets** provide the essential content needed during the shorter rotations. They will also provide the basic content needed for USMLE Steps 2 and 3. Or, if you were unable to fit in the rotation, these new pocket-sized **Blueprints** are just what you need.

Each book will focus on the high-yield essential content for the most commonly encountered problems of the specialty. Each book features these special appendices:

- Career and residency opportunities
- Commonly prescribed medications
- Self-test Q&A section

Ask for these at your medical bookstore or check them out online at www.lww.com.

Blueprints Dermatology
Blueprints Urology
Blueprints Pediatric Infectious Diseases
Blueprints Ophthalmology
Blueprints Plastic Surgery
Blueprints Orthopedics
Blueprints Hematology and Oncology
Blueprints Infectious Diseases
Blueprints Anesthesiology

BLUEPRINTS Pocket Gastroenterology

Shilpa Grover, MD
Gastroenterology Fellow
Department of Internal Medicine
Division of Gastroenterology
Brigham & Women's Hospital
Boston, Massachusetts

Wolters Kluwer Health | Lippincott Williams & Wilkins
Philadelphia • Baltimore • New York • London
Buenos Aires • Hong Kong • Sydney • Tokyo

Acquisitions Editor: Donna M. Balado
Managing Editor: Stacey L. Sebring
Marketing Manager: Jennifer Kuklinski
Production Editor: Jennifer D.W. Glazer
Designer: Doug Smock
Compositor: International Typesetting and Composition
Printer: R.R. Donnelley & Sons—Crawfordsville

351 West Camden Street
Baltimore, MD 21201

530 Walnut Street
Philadelphia, PA 19106

The publisher is not responsible (as a matter of product liability, negligence, or otherwise) for any injury resulting from any material contained herein. This publication contains information relating to general principles of medical care that should not be construed as specific instructions for individual patients. Manufacturers' product information and package inserts should be reviewed for current information, including contraindications, dosages, and precautions.

Printed in the United States of America

Library of Congress Cataloging-in-Publication Data

Grover, Shilpa.
Blueprints pocket gastroenterology / Shilpa Grover.
p. ; cm. — (Blueprints for your pocket!)
Includes bibliographical references and index.
ISBN-13: 978-1-4051-0470-8
ISBN-10: 1-4051-0470-8
1. Gastroenterology—Handbooks, manuals, etc. 2. Digestive organs—Diseases—Handbooks, manuals, etc. I. Title. II. Series.
[DNLM: 1. Digestive System Diseases—Handbooks. WI 39 G883b 2007]
RC802.G76 2007
616.3'3—dc22

2006026469

The publishers have made every effort to trace the copyright holders for borrowed material. If they have inadvertently overlooked any, they will be pleased to make the necessary arrangements at the first opportunity.

To purchase additional copies of this book, call our customer service department at **(800) 638-3030** or fax orders to **(301) 223-2320.** International customers should call **(301) 223-2300.**

Visit Lippincott Williams & Wilkins on the Internet: http://www.LWW.com. Lippincott Williams & Wilkins customer service representatives are available from 8:30 am to 6:00 pm, EST.

06 07 08 09 10
1 2 3 4 5 6 7 8 9 10

To my family

Preface

Blueprints have become the standard for medical students to use during their clerkship rotations and subinternships and as a review book for taking the USMLE Steps 2 and 3.

Blueprints initially were only available for the five main specialties: medicine, pediatrics, obstetrics and gynecology, surgery, and psychiatry. Students found these books so valuable that they asked for **Blueprints** in other topics, and so gastroenterology, family medicine, emergency medicine, neurology, cardiology, and radiology were added.

In an effort to answer a need for high-yield review books for the elective rotations, Lippincott Williams & Wilkins now bring you **Blueprints** in pocket size. These books are developed to provide students in the shorter, elective rotations, often taken in 4th year, with the same high yield, essential contents of the larger **Blueprint** books. These new pocket-sized **Blueprints** will be invaluable for those students who need to know the essentials of a clinical area but were unable to take the rotation. Students in physician assistant, nurse practitioner, and osteopath programs will find these books meet their needs for the clinical specialties.

Feedback from student reviewers gives high praise for this addition to the **Blueprint** brand. Each of these new books was developed to be read in a short time and to address the basics needed during a particular clinical rotation. Please see the Series Page for a list of the books that will soon be in your bookstore.

Acknowledgments

I would like to express my gratitude to Drs. Joel Katz, Bruce Levy, and Marc Sabatine for their enthusiastic support of this endeavor. I am grateful to Drs. Norton Greenberger and Allen Kachalia for their advice and contribution.

I would also like to acknowledge Dr. Kevin Sheth, Kate Heinle and Beverly Copland for their suggestions and recommendations. Thanks also to Betty Sun, Donna Balado, Kathleen Scogna and Stacey Sebring at Lippincott Williams & Wilkins. I am also extremely grateful to Dr. Katherine Black for her encouragement.

Finally, I'd like to thank my family for their patience and unwavering support.

Contents

Chapter 1

Anatomy of the Gastrointestinal Tract

Esophagus

Surgical Anatomy

The esophagus, located in the posterior mediastinum, extends from the cricopharyngeal sphincter to the stomach. The esophagus is located posterior to the trachea, anterior to the vertebral column, and is flanked laterally by the aorta on the left and by the pleura bilaterally. The lower end of the esophagus is an important site for portosystemic anastomosis. In patients with portal hypertension, these anastomoses dilate and form esophageal varices.

Histology

The esophageal wall consists of four layers. (a) The mucosa is the innermost layer and consists of stratified squamous nonkeratinized epithelium that transitions to columnar epithelium near the gastroesophageal junction; (b) the muscularis mucosa consists of striated muscle in the upper one third and smooth muscle in the lower two thirds; (c) the submucosa consists of mucus-secreting glands; and (d) the adventitia is the outermost layer consisting of connective tissue.

Blood Supply and Lymphatic Drainage

The upper esophagus is supplied by the superior and inferior thyroid arteries, and the lower esophagus is supplied by the intercostal, left gastric, and phrenic arteries. Venous drainage of the upper esophagus is via the inferior thyroid and vertebral veins. The mid and lower esophagus are drained by the azygous, hemiazygous, and left gastric veins. The lymphatic drainage of the esophagus enters the cervical, mediastinal, gastric and celiac lymph nodes.

Nerve Supply

Parasympathetic innervation is via the vagus nerve; sympathetic nerve supply is via the greater splanchnic nerve.

Stomach

Surgical Anatomy

The stomach is divided anatomically into the fundus, body, antrum, and pylorus. The fundus is the superior part of the stomach;

the body extends from the fundus to the angle of the stomach (incisura angularis); and the antrum extends from the body to the pylorus.

Histology

The stomach consists of the following layers: (a) mucosa consisting of columnar epithelium with mucus-secreting cells, (b) muscularis mucosa consisting of smooth muscle, (c) submucosa containing the Meissner plexus, (d) muscularis externa with inner circular and outer longitudinal muscle, in addition to the myenteric plexus and (e) the outermost serosa. The cardia of the stomach has special cells that secrete mucus. Fundic parietal cells secrete hydrochloric acid and intrinsic factor, and chief cells secrete pepsinogen. The antrum contains G cells, which produce gastrin.

Blood Supply and Lymphatic Drainage

Left and right gastric arteries are located along the lesser curvature, left and right gastroepiploic arteries on the greater curvature. The short gastric artery supplies the fundus, and the gastroduodenal artery supplies the pylorus. Veins of the stomach drain into the portal, superior mesenteric, and splenic veins. Lymphatics drain into regional lymph nodes and then into the celiac lymph nodes.

Nerve Supply

The stomach has sympathetic and parasympathetic innervation. Sympathetic nerves are derived from T6–T10 via the greater splanchnic nerve and the celiac and hepatic plexus. Parasympathetic innervation is via the vagus nerve through the esophageal plexus and the gastric nerve. Parasympathetic stimulation is secretomotor and motor; sympathetic stimulation is vasomotor and motor to the pyloric sphincter (Figs. 1-1 and 1-2).

SMALL INTESTINE

Duodenum

Surgical Anatomy

The duodenum is divided into four parts. The first part extends from the pylorus to meet the second or descending part of the duodenum at the superior duodenal flexure. The second part of the duodenum extends from the superior to the inferior duodenal flexure. The ampulla of Vater, through which the common bile duct and the

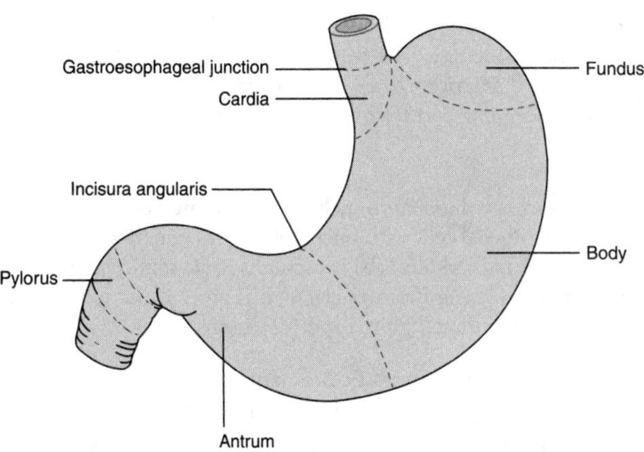

Figure 1-1 • Anatomy of the stomach. (From Karp S, Morris J, Soybel, D. *Blueprints surgery.* 3rd ed. Oxford: Blackwell; 2004, with permission.)

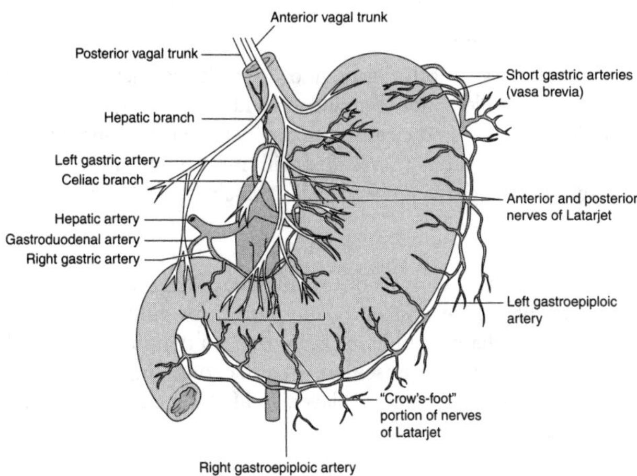

Figure 1-2 • Blood supply and parasympathetic innervation of the stomach and duodenum. (From Karp S, Morris J, Soybel, D. *Blueprints surgery.* 3rd ed. Oxford: Blackwell; 2004, with permission.)

pancreatic duct drain, is located on the medial wall of the second part of the duodenum. The third or transverse part of the duodenum is related anteriorly to the superior mesenteric vessels, and the fourth or ascending part terminates at the ligament of Treitz.

Histology

The layers of the duodenum include: (a) the mucosa consisting of columnar epithelial cells with microvilli and invaginations that form the crypts of Lieberkühn; (b) muscularis mucosa; (c) submucosa with mucus-secreting Brunner glands that are specific to the duodenum; (d) muscularis externa and (e) the serosa.

Blood Supply and Lymphatic Drainage

The duodenum is supplied by the superior and inferior pancreaticoduodenal arteries. Venous drainage is via the splenic and superior mesenteric veins. Lymph from the duodenum drains into the pancreaticoduodenal lymph nodes and hepatic nodes and ultimately into the celiac lymph nodes.

Nerve Supply

Sympathetic innervation via T9–T10, and parasympathetic supply is via the vagus nerve.

Jejunum and Ileum

Surgical Anatomy

The jejunum begins at the ligament of Treitz. It has thick walls, large mucosal folds called plicae semilunaris, and is characterized by long vasa rectae. There is no clear distinction between the jejunum and the ileum. The ileum is thin walled with more abundant fat in the mesentery and is characterized by short vasa recta and plicae.

Histology

The small intestine consists of the following layers: (a) the innermost layer of the jejunum and ileum formed by villi; (b) the submucosa of the ileum containing collections of lymphocytes called Peyer patches; (c) the muscularis externa consisting of an inner circular and outer longitudinal layer, and (d) the outermost layer, the serosa.

Blood Supply and Lymphatic Drainage

Arterial supply and venous drainage of the jejunum and ileum are via the superior mesenteric artery and vein. Lymphatics drain into the wall of jejunum and ileum and then into the nodes along the superior mesenteric artery.

Nerve Supply

The submucosa contains the nerve plexus of Meissner; the muscularis contains the nerve plexus of Auerbach.

LARGE INTESTINE

Colon

Surgical Anatomy

The colon is approximately 1.5 m in length, extending from the ileocecal junction to the anus, and is divided into the cecum, ascending colon, transverse colon, descending colon, sigmoid, rectum, and anal canal. Fat-filled collections of peritoneum called appendices epiploica are located on the outer surface of the colon. These appendices occasionally become inflamed and cause acute abdominal pain, a condition referred to as appendagitis epipolica.

Histology

The colon consists of the following layers: (a) the innermost layer consisting of columnar epithelium-lined mucosa; (b) the muscularis mucosa; (c) the submucosa; (d) the muscularis externa consisting of inner circular and a thin outer longitudinal layer that forms three bands called taenia coli; (e) and the outermost adventitia.

Blood Supply and Lymphatic Drainage

The superior mesenteric artery, through the ilocolic, right, and middle colic artery, supplies the cecum to the splenic flexure. The inferior mesenteric artery, through the left colic, sigmoid, and superior rectal branches, supplies the descending colon, sigmoid, and upper rectum. Venous drainage is via the superior and inferior mesenteric veins. Lymphatics from the colon drain into the following lymph nodes: epicolic lymph nodes on the wall of the colon; paracolic lymph nodes around the medial wall of the ascending and descending colon and mesocolic border of the transverse colon; intermediate lymph nodes along the main branches of vessels supplying the colon; and terminal lymph nodes along superior and inferior mesenteric arteries.

Nerve Supply

Parasympathetic innervation of the colon derived from the midgut (cecum, appendix, ascending colon, and the right two thirds of the transverse colon) is via the vagus nerve, and sympathetic innervation is from T11–L1 from the celiac and superior mesenteric ganglia. The colon derived from the hindgut (left one third of the transverse colon, descending colon, sigmoid colon, and proximal rectum) receives parasympathetic innervation from the pelvic splanchnic nerve through superior hypogastric and inferior mesenteric plexi, and sympathetic innervation is from the lumbar sympathetic chain L1–L2.

Rectum

Surgical Anatomy

The rectum extends from the sigmoid colon to the anal canal.

Histology

The layers of the rectum are as follows: (a) mucosa consisting of columnar epithelium with numerous goblet cells; (b) the submucosa containing nerve plexi; (c) the muscularis externa; and (d) the outermost serosa/adventitia.

Blood Supply and Lymphatic Drainage

The upper two thirds of the rectum is supplied by the superior rectal branch of the inferior mesenteric artery and the middle rectal of the internal iliac artery; the lower one third is supplied by the inferior rectal a branch of the pudendal artery. Venous drainage of the upper two thirds is via the superior and middle rectal veins, which in turn drain into the inferior mesenteric vein, and the drainage of the lower one third enters the inferior rectal veins, which in turn drain into the inferior vena cava (IVC). Lymphatics from the upper two thirds drain into the inferior mesenteric lymph nodes, and from the lower one third drain into the inferior mesenteric and internal iliac nodes.

Nerve Supply

Sympathetic innervation of the rectum is from L1, L2; parasympathetic innervation (S2, S3, S4) is through the superior rectal or inferior mesenteric and inferior hypogastric plexi.

Anal Canal

The anal canal extends from the anorectal junction to the anus and is 3.8 cm in length.

Histology

The upper 15 mm of the anal canal is stratified columnar epithelium. The mucous membrane forms vertical folds called the anal columns of Morgagni. The lower ends of the anal columns form anal valves. The anal valves together form a transverse line around the anal canal called the pectinate line. The pectinate line represents the junction of the ectodermal and endodermal parts of the anal canal. The middle 15 mm is stratified squamous epithelium, and the lower 8 mm is stratified squamous epithelium with sweat glands and hair follicles. The anal canal is surrounded by the circular muscle that forms the internal anal sphincter, which is involuntary. The external anal sphincter consists of striated muscle and is voluntary. The longitudinal muscle of the rectum fuses with the puborectalis at the anorectal junction and extends between the internal and external sphincters.

Blood Supply and Lymphatic Drainage

The anal canal is supplied by the superior and inferior rectal arteries. The submucosal internal rectal venous plexus drains into the superior rectal vein and communicates with the external plexus formed by the middle and inferior rectal veins. The internal plexus is an important site for portosystemic anastomosis, and dilatation of these veins results in internal hemorrhoids. The external rectal plexus is drained by the superior rectal vein, which drains into the inferior mesenteric vein; by the middle rectal vein, which drains into the internal iliac vein; and by the inferior rectal vein.

Nerve Supply

The anal canal above the pectinate line receives sympathetic innervation from the inferior hypogastric plexus (L1, L2) and parasympathetic innervation through the pelvic splanchnic nerves S2, S3, S4. The part of the anal canal below the pectinate line is supplied by somatic nerves through the inferior rectal nerve (S2, S3, S4). The internal anal sphincter is involuntary and contracts in response to parasympathetic stimulation. The external anal sphincter is voluntary and is supplied by the inferior rectal nerve and the perineal branch of the fourth sacral nerve.

Liver

Surgical Anatomy

The liver can be is divided into eight segments based on the blood supply and biliary drainage. The portal fissure that extends from the left side of the gallbladder fossa to the left side of the IVC divides the liver into the physiologic right and left lobes. Segment I is the caudate lobe of the liver; segments II–IV form the left lobe; and segments V–VIII form the right lobe of the liver (Fig. 1-3).

Histology

The hepatic lobule consists of radiating hepatocytes and sinusoids from the central vein. Sinusoids are lined by endothelial cells, and Kupffer cells (intrahepatocytic macrophages) are attached to the endothelial surface.

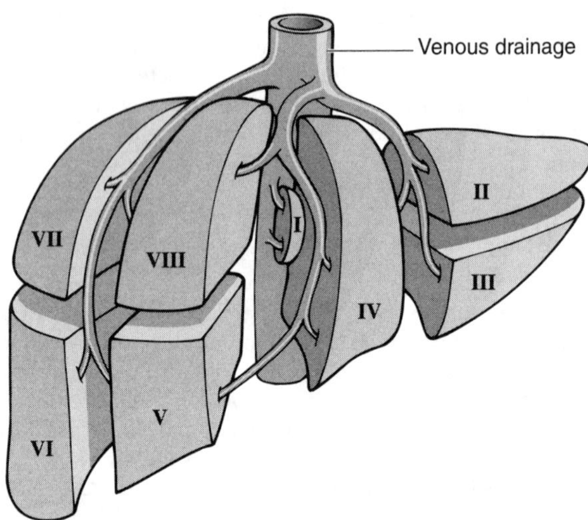

Figure 1-3 • Segmental anatomy of the liver. (From Karp S, Morris J, Soybel, D. *Blueprints surgery.* 3rd ed. Oxford: Blackwell; 2004, with permission.)

Portal triads located at the periphery of the lobule consist of a hepatic arteriole, bile ductule, and portal venule.

Blood Supply and Lymphatic Drainage

The portal vein provides 80% of the blood supply. The common hepatic artery, a branch of the celiac artery, provides 20% of the blood supply. Venous drainage of the liver is via the hepatic veins, which are arranged in two groups. The upper group consists of the right and left hepatic veins, which drain into the IVC, and the middle hepatic vein, which drains into the left hepatic vein. The lower group consists of veins from the caudate lobe and the right lobe of the liver and drain directly into the IVC.

Nerve Supply

Both sympathetic and parasympathetic innervation of the liver is via the hepatic plexus.

Gallbladder and Biliary Tract (Fig. 1-4)

Surgical Anatomy

The biliary tree consists of the right and left hepatic ducts, which join to form the common hepatic duct. The gallbladder consists of a fundus, body, infundibulum, and neck. The cystic duct drains

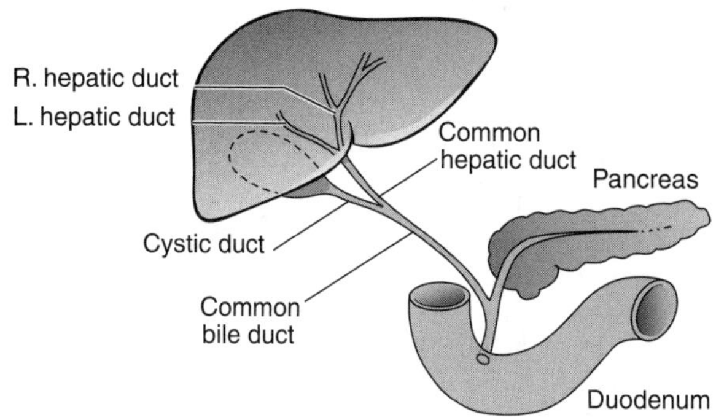

Figure 1-4 • Gallbladder and biliary tree. (From Karp S, Morris J, Soybel, D. *Blueprints surgery.* 3rd ed. Oxford: Blackwell; 2004, with permission.)

the gallbladder and joins the common hepatic duct to form the common bile duct. The common bile duct joins the pancreatic duct to form the common channel that leads into the ampulla of Vater in the medial wall of the second part of the duodenum. The sphincter of Oddi is smooth muscle around the common bile duct and pancreatic duct.

Histology

The layers of the gallbladder include: (a) the mucosa consisting of columnar epithelium with characteristic Rokitansky–Aschoff sinuses in the wall, (b) a muscular layer, and (c) the adventitia. Ducts of Luschka are microscopic ducts that are present in 1% of the population and directly drain from the liver to the gallbladder.

Blood Supply and Lymphatic Drainage

The cystic artery, which is usually derived from the right hepatic artery, is the main source of blood supply to the gallbladder, the cystic and hepatic duct, and the upper part of the bile duct. Branches of the superior pancreaticoduodenal artery supply the lower part of the bile duct. The superior surface of the gallbladder is drained by veins through the gallbladder fossa into hepatic veins; the remainder of the gallbladder is drained by the cystic vein, which then drains into the liver. Lymphatic drainage of the gallbladder follows the veins and enters the cystic lymph node and the hepatic lymph nodes.

Nerve Supply

Sympathetic innervation is from the cystic plexus of nerves derived from the celiac plexus, and parasympathetic supply is from the vagus nerve.

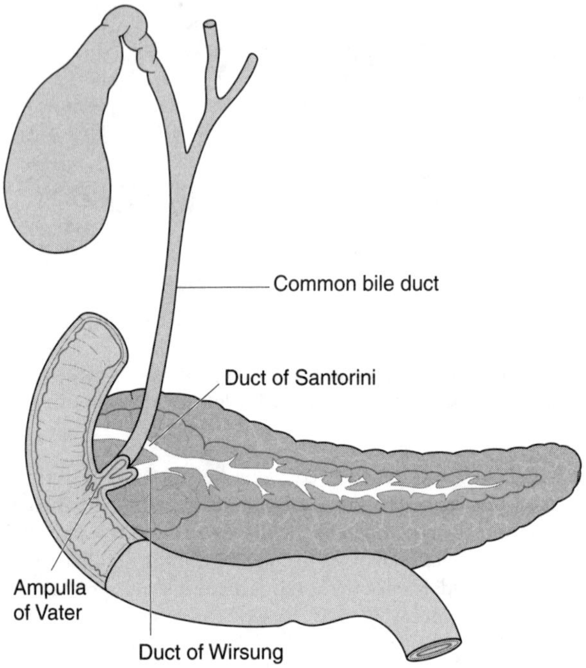

Figure 1-5 • The pancreatic ductal system including the ducts of Wirsung (major duct) and Santorini (minor duct). (From Karp S, Morris J, Soybel, D. *Blueprints surgery.* 3rd ed. Oxford: Blackwell; 2004, with permission.)

Pancreas (Fig. 1-5)

Surgical Anatomy

The pancreas, a retroperitoneal organ with endocrine and exocrine function, is divided into the head, neck, body, and tail. The main pancreatic duct of Wirsung begins at the tail of the pancreas. As it traverses the body and head of the pancreas, it is joined by numerous branches giving it a herringbone appearance. In the head of the pancreas, the main pancreatic duct joins the common bile duct to form the hepatopancreatic ampulla of Vater. The ampulla opens into the major duodenal papilla on the medial wall of the second part of the duodenum. The accessory pancreatic duct of Santorini traverses the head of the pancreas and drains into the minor duodenal papilla.

Histology

Exocrine cells: Acinar cells produce the pancreatic enzymes elastase, phospholipase, amylase, lipase, trypsin, and chymotrypsin. Ductal cells produce bicarbonate in response to secretin.

Endocrine cells: Alpha cells produce glucagon; beta cells produce insulin; delta cells produce somatostatin, and F cells produce pancreatic polypeptide.

Blood Supply and Lymphatic Drainage

The head of the pancreas is supplied by the anterior and posterior pancreaticoduodenal arteries. The proximal body is supplied by the superior and inferior pancreatic arteries, and the distal body and tail are supplied by the splenic, gastroepiploic, and dorsal pancreatic arteries. Venous drainage of the pancreas is into the superior mesenteric and splenic veins, which in turn drain into the portal vein. Lymphatic drainage of the pancreas follows the vascular supply and enters the celiac and superior mesenteric lymph nodes.

Nerve Supply

Parasympathetic nerve supply to the pancreas is provided by the vagus nerve and sympathetic innervation by the splanchnic plexus. Parasympathetic nerves are secretory; sympathetic innervation is vasomotor.

Chapter

2 Gastroenterological Emergencies

Upper Gastrointestinal Bleeding

Incidence/Etiology

Upper gastrointestinal (GI) bleeding is estimated to be responsible for 5% of emergency room visits per year and has an associated mortality of 6% to 8% (Table 2-1).

Clinical Manifestations

Upper GI bleeding can manifest as hematemesis with vomiting of bright red blood or coffee-ground material formed by the conversion of hemoglobin to hematin by gastric acid. Alternatively, patients may have melena with the passage of dark tarry stool; in rare cases massive upper GI bleeding can result in the passage of bright red blood per rectum. In a retrospective study by Witting et al. of patients admitted to an emergency room for GI bleeding without hematemesis, the presence of black stool, age less than 50 years and BUN/Creatinine ≥ predicted an upper GI source of bleeding.

History

- Duration of the GI bleed and extent
- Prior history of GI bleeding
- Nonsteroidal anti-inflammatory drug (NSAID) use
- Liver disease and the presence of varices
- Prior colonoscopy/esophagogastroduodenoscopy (EGD)
- Known diverticular disease, hemorrhoids
- Recent polypectomy
- Coagulopathy from anticoagulation
- Comorbid illnesses
- Associated symptoms: Abdominal pain, nausea, vomiting, chest pain, shortness of breath, lightheadedness, palpitations

Physical Examination

- Assess degree of volume loss with the degree of tachycardia and hypotension
- Stigmata of liver disease: Scleral icterus, spider nevi, gynecomastia, parotid enlargement, ascites, caput medusa
- Rectal exam

TABLE 2-1 Causes of Upper GI Bleeding

Cause	%
Peptic ulcer disease	55%
Esophageal varices	14%
Arteriovenous malformations	6%
Mallory–Weiss tear	5%
Tumors	4%
Dieulafoy lesions, gastric antral vascular ectasia, aorto enteric fistula	1%

Data from Jutabha R et al. *Med Clin North Am.* 1996;80(5):1035–1068.

- Nasogastric lavage to determine if there is an upper or lower gastrointestinal bleeding source

Management

- Keep the patient NPO (nil per oral)
- Airway protection: Intubation may be necessary in patients with upper GI bleed who are unable to protect their airway due to altered mental status or massive hematemesis.
- Access: All patients with GI bleeding should have adequate intravenous access for fluid resuscitation with the placement of two large-bore (16- to 18-gauge) peripheral intravenous lines or large-bore central venous line.
- Volume resuscitation: Intravenous fluid resuscitation with normal saline. Blood transfusions with transfusion goals in accordance with the patient's comorbidity; fresh frozen plasma/ phytonadione to reverse coagulopathy may be necessary.
- Monitoring: Tachycardia and hypotension are signs of significant blood loss; such patients should have continuous hemodynamic monitoring.
- Acid suppression in nonvariceal upper GI bleeding:
  - H2 Blockers: A study by Walt et al. of acid suppression with continuous infusion of an H2 blocker famotidine in patients with nonvariceal upper GI bleeding showed that, in patients with peptic ulcers with high risk stigmata, H2 blockers did not appear to significantly affect rebleeding, the need for surgery, or mortality.
  - Proton pump inhibitors (PPI): By inhibiting the parietal cell H-K ATPase and therefore gastric acid production, PPI (oral or intravenous) have been shown in multiple studies to be more effective than H2 blockers in decreasing ulcer, rebleeding, and the need for surgery. They have not been shown to decrease mortality. It may be reasonable to treat patients with high-risk stigmata on EGD, such as adherent clot and visible vessel, with intravenous PPI for 72 h and then an oral PPI. Patients without such stigmata on EGD can be treated with an oral PPI.

- Upper endoscopy: EGD is essential in detecting the source of bleeding and has the advantage that it is a relatively safe procedure that provides therapeutic options and helps predict the chances of rebleeding. In patients with variceal bleeding, sclerotherapy or variceal band ligation can be performed to control bleeding.
- Octreotide: Infusions for 5 days in patients with variceal bleeding can cause a decrease in portal pressure that is short lived. However, octreotide also inhibits the release of glucagon, which increases portal pressure postprandially and a decrease in the rebound in pressure that occurs after the correction of hypovolemia. There may also be a role for octreotide in patients with nonvariceal GI bleeding.
- Vasopressin: Reduces splanchnic blood flow and portal pressure, but causes systemic vasoconstriction and myocardial and mesenteric ischemia/infarction. Given these side effects, the use of vasopressin is therefore very limited.
- *Helicobacter pylori* testing: Infection with *H. pylori* has been shown to be an independent risk factor for rebleeding. Patients should therefore be tested and treated if positive. If negative, a confirmatory test should be performed given the possibility of false-negative results in the setting of an acute bleed.
- In patients with variceal bleeding in whom endoscopy fails, management options include:
  - Repeat attempt at endoscopic therapy.
  - Balloon tamponade is useful in patients following failure of endoscopic therapy. Airway protection with intubation is necessary prior to insertion of the balloon. The high risk of complications including esophageal rupture and rebleeding following deflation of the balloon limits the utility of balloon tamponade to a temporizing measure.
- Transjugular intrahepatic portosystemic shunt (TIPS) involves the placement of a catheter via the internal jugular vein into the intrahepatic portion of the hepatic vein. The shunt thereby creates a low-resistance path between the hepatic vein and the portal vein and acts as a side-to-side portocaval shunt. TIPS is the procedure of choice in patients with recurrent bleeding, patients who are poor surgical candidates, and as a bridge to transplant in patients with advanced liver disease. Hepatic encephalopathy, infection, bleeding, and stenosis of the shunt are potential complications.
- Surgery: Should be considered in patients with recurrent variceal bleeding when TIPS is not available or is not technically feasible. In such cases, esophageal staple transection with or without esophagogastric devascularization or a portosystemic shunt procedure can be performed, but both procedures carry a high morbidity and mortality in patients with advanced liver disease.

TABLE 2-2 Risk of Recurrent Bleeding According to Endoscopic Stigmata

Clean base	<3%
Flat spot	<8%
Adherent clot	30–35%
Visible vessel	50%
Active bleed	Approaches 100%

Jensen DM. Spots and clots—leave them or treat them? Why and how to treat. *Canadian J Gastroenterol* 1999;13,413–415.
Savides and Jensen DM. Therapeutic endoscopy for nonvariceal gastrointestinal bleeding, *Gastroenterol Clin N Amer* 2000;29:465–487.
Johnson GH. Gastrointestinal Endoscopy, 1990; 316–320.

Prognosis

- Bleeding stops spontaneously without recurrence in 80% of cases of nonvariceal upper GI bleeding; 20% of patients rebleed. The risk of recurrent bleeding has been strongly associated with stigmata on endoscopy (Table 2-2).
- Scoring systems, such as the Rockall risk score, that include age, presence of shock, comorbidity, diagnosis, and endoscopic stigmata have been used to predict the risk of recurrent bleeding. Each factor is assigned a score of 0 to 3 with a maximum score of 11. Patients are considered at low risk for rebleeding if the Rockall score ≤2.

Lower Gastrointestinal Bleeding

Lower GI bleeding is defined as bleeding distal to the ligament of Treitz (jejunum, ileum, and colon).

Incidence/Etiology

Studies have estimated an annual incidence of 20.5/100,000 with an increase in incidence with age (Table 2-3).

Clinical Manifestations

Hematochezia with the passage of bright red blood or dark blood and clots suggests a lower GI source of bleeding. It is important to perform a nasogastric lavage in patients with GI bleeding as studies have shown that 10% to 15% patients with hematochezia have an upper GI bleed and one third of patients with lower GI bleed can have melena. A nasogastric tube can also be of assistance in rapid preparation of the bowel for colonoscopy.

TABLE 2-3 Sources of Lower GI Bleeding

Diverticulosis	30%
Anorectal (Hemorrhoids, fissure, ulcer)	16%
Ischemia	10%
Colitis	8%
Post polypectomy	7%
Malignancy	6%
Angiodysplasia	3%
IBD	4%
Unknown	9%
Other	5%

Strate et al. Timing of colonscopy: impact of length of hospital stay in patients with acute lower gastrointestinal bleeding. *Am J Gastroenterol* 2003;98:317–322.

Management

- Intravenous access: Adequate intravenous access with two large-bore peripheral intravenous catheters or a cordis central venous catheter to allow large-volume resuscitation.
- Fluid resuscitation: As with any case of GI bleeding, the first task is to perform adequate fluid resuscitation. Blood transfusions to maintain the hematocrit above a certain target should be based on the patient's comorbidities. Coagulopathy (international normalized ratio, INR > 1.5) or thrombocytopenia (platelets < 50,000) may need to be corrected.
- Colonoscopy: Enables localization of the source of bleeding and allows for biopsies to be taken and therapeutic interventions to be performed. Rapid bowel preparation with the use of 6 L of polyethylene glycol enables an urgent colonoscopy (within 12 h) to be performed. Colonoscopy has a high diagnostic and therapeutic yield but has the disadvantage of the need for time to prepare the bowel.
- Nuclear imaging: Detects bleeding at the rate of 0.1 to 0.5 cc/min. A tagged red cell scan is a relatively inexpensive and noninvasive diagnostic test. The disadvantages include limited accuracy due to the movement of blood, lack of therapeutic benefit, and because it is used in conjunction with angiography, bleeding may stop in the time interval between the two tests.
- Angiography: Should be performed if bleeding is occurring at a rate of 0.5 to 1 cc/min. The advantages of angiography are that is does not require bowel preparation, that the localization of the source is accurate, and that it can be therapeutic with the use of embolization. Disadvantages include limited diagnostic yield and a high rate of complications, which include renal failure, arterial

embolization resulting in infarction, bleeding, thrombosis, vasopressin-induced ischemia, and arrhythmias.
- Push enteroscopy: Indicated in patients with continued bleeding if the site cannot be identified after an EGD or colonoscopy to visualize the proximal jejunum, which may be the site of bleeding.
- Surgery: Indicated in cases of recurrent bleeding following failed endoscopy and angiography.

Diarrhea

Diarrhea is defined as an increase in stool frequency greater than or equal to three stools in a 24-h period of less-than-normal form and consistency. Diarrhea that occurs for <4 weeks duration is acute; diarrhea is defined as chronic if it lasts >4 weeks.

Major Causes of Acute Diarrhea

Infectious

- Viral: Rotavirus, Adenovirus, Norwalk, Corona, Calcivirus
- Bacterial:
  - Preformed toxins: *Bacillus cereus, Staphylococcus aureus, Clostridium perfringens*
  - Noninvasive (nonbloody diarrhea): Enterotoxin producing: enterotoxigenic *Escherichia coli, Vibrio cholerae*; cytotoxin producing: *E. coli* O157:H7, *C. difficile*
  - Invasive bacteria (bloody diarrhea): *Salmonella, Shigella, Campylobacter, E. coli* O157:H7, *Clostridium difficile, Yersinia*
  - Parasitic: *Entamoeba histolytica, Giardia, Cryptosporidium, Microsporidium, Cyclospora*

Noninfectious

- Dietary: Nonabsorbable sugars
- Medications
- Fecal impaction
- Ischemic colitis

Clinical Manifestations

- It is important to determine the onset, duration, frequency, stool characteristics such as the presence of blood or mucus, abdominal pain, associated fever, and to assess the degree of dehydration.
- Historical clues that may help in determining the cause of diarrhea: Prior episodes of diarrhea; weight loss; age-appropriate endoscopic evaluation; recent camping/travel; food history; medication use including antibiotics, laxatives, chemotherapy, and over-the-counter supplements; sick contacts; immunosuppression due to HIV infection with CD4 count, organ transplantation;

heat/cold intolerance suggestive of thyroid disease; wheezing and bronchospasm suggestive of carcinoid syndrome; family history of inflammatory bowel disease (IBD), polyps, cancer.

- Most cases of diarrhea are self-limited and mild. Cases of diarrhea that merit further evaluation are as follows:
  - Bloody diarrhea
  - Dehydration secondary to the diarrhea
  - Severe abdominal pain
  - Duration >48 h and more than six unformed stools in 24 h
  - Fever >101°F
  - Diarrhea in elderly individuals
  - Immunocompromised patient (HIV, chemotherapy, on steroids or immunosuppressants)
  - Recent antibiotic use or hospitalization

Clinical Manifestations of Specific Pathogens and Complications

- *Campylobacter jejuni:* Remains the leading cause of diarrhea (4% to 11% of cases). *Campylobacter* is associated with late-onset complications that occur 1 to 2 weeks following an infection:
  - Reactive arthritis: Patients may have associated conjunctivitis with arthritis that typically involves the knees, ankles, wrists, small joints of the hands that lasts for weeks-months and then resolves spontaneously.
  - Guillain–Barré syndrome (GBS): *Campylobacter* infection is responsible for one third of cases of GBS. It is hypothesized that GBS results from a molecular mimicry whereby antibodies to *Campylobacter* cross-react with GM1 ganglioside present in nerve myelin. Studies have shown that *Campylobacter*-associated GBS has worse outcomes than GBS associated with other infections.
- *Salmonella* gastroenteritis
  - The source of *Salmonella* is usually contaminated eggs.
  - Typhoid fever is caused by *S. typhi* or *S. paratyphi*.
  - Patients have high-grade persistent fever with relative bradycardia, malaise, anorexia, nausea, hepatosplenomegaly, rose spots (erythematous, blanching maculopapular rash) on the chest and abdomen.
  - Laboratory studies are remarkable for a leukocytosis with predominant mononuclear cells. Liver function tests can be elevated two to three times the upper limit of normal.

Diagnosis

- Stool fecal leukocytes: Detected by Wright stain (less sensitive) or the lactoferrin assay (more sensitive and specific). Stool fecal leukocytes help differentiate inflammatory from noninflammatory diarrhea.

- Occult blood: The presence of occult blood and fecal leukocytes favors the presence of a bacterial pathogen as the cause of diarrhea.
- *Clostridium difficile* toxin: *C. difficile* infection should be suspected in patients with recent antibiotic use in the last 14 days and nosocomial. Stool cytotoxicity assay is the gold standard with 94% sensitivity and 99% specificity. Enzyme-linked immunosorbent assay (ELISA) for *C. difficile* has lower sensitivity (75% to 90%) and comparable specificity (99%). The ELISA for *C. difficile* is a more rapid assay but tests only for toxin A (enterotoxin); patients with toxin B infections will test negative even though they have a *C. difficile* infection.
- Stool for ova and parasites: Three specimens need to be tested for ova and parasites due to intermittent shedding. Testing is indicated in patients with recent travel abroad, camping, immunocompromised hosts or patient with diarrhea for >2 weeks. Infections with Giardia and cryptosporidium are commonly associated with camping due to exposure to untreated water.
- Stool cultures: Indicated in patients with bloody diarrhea, patients with inflammatory bowel disease, immunocompromised patients, and in food handlers.
- Endoscopy: Indicated in acute diarrhea in patients with bloody diarrhea where infection needs to be differentiated from IBD, in diarrhea in immunocompromised patients where stool cultures have limited sensitivity and definitive diagnosis can only be made by endoscopy with biopsy. Cytomegalovirus (CMV) colitis, which is often right sided necessitates a colonoscopy as CMV antigenemia does not necessarily indicate colitis. In patients with *Clostridium difficile*, flexible sigmoidoscopy shows yellow-white pseudomembranes.

Treatment

- Supportive care with oral rehydration solution: Oral rehydration solutions containing sodium chloride, potassium chloride, sodium bicarbonate, and glucose should be used in preference to solutions that replace sweat loss.
- Lifestyle modification: Lactose intolerance is common following acute gastroenteritis and therefore lactose-containing products should be temporarily avoided. Sugar substitutes can cause osmotic diarrhea and should be avoided. There are no data to support specific dietary recommendations. Medications should be reviewed.
- Probiotics: Recolonizing the gut with normal flora has been used in cases of traveler's diarrhea to shorten the course and decrease severity.

- Antidiarrheal agents: Diphenoxylate and loperamide decrease the motility of the bowel and should be used with extreme caution given the possibility of toxic megacolon.
- Antibiotics: In patients with suspected *C. difficile* diarrhea, it is appropriate to start empiric metronidazole after stool has been sent for *C. difficile* toxin. In patients with fever, symptoms for >1 week, and more than eight stools per day or in an immunocompromised host, it is appropriate to treat empirically with a fluoroquinolone. However, in patients with suspected enterohemorrhagic *E. coli* (*EHEC*), antibiotics should be avoided as there is concern that it may precipitate hemolytic uremic syndrome (HUS).

Chronic Diarrhea

Diarrhea for >4 weeks is defined as chronic diarrhea.

History

- Characteristics of diarrhea: Onset, duration, and frequency.
- Improvement of symptoms with fasting: Suggests a malabsorptive cause of diarrhea; secretory diarrhea persists even with fasting.
- Timing in relation to food: Carbohydrate malabsorption occurs 1 to 2 h after a meal; irritable bowel syndrome is also aggravated by eating.
- Nocturnal symptoms: Suggest an organic pathology.
- Excess flatulence: Suggests carbohydrate malabsorption.
- Weight loss: Seen with malabsorption and malignancy.
- Associated symptoms: Flushing, sweating, and bronchospasm suggest carcinoid syndrome.
- Medications: Use of antacids, antibiotics, immunosuppressants, and steroids should be determined.
- Diet: Lactose, sugar substitutes, and olestra can be associated with diarrhea.
- Race: Celiac sprue is more common in patients of northern European descent.
- Surgeries Bowel resection (bacterial overgrowth and short gut syndrome).
- Travel history: Parasitic infestations and tropical sprue.
- Past medical history: Anemia (celiac disease), radiation exposure (radiation enteritis), recurrent ulcers (Zollinger–Ellison syndrome), diabetes (poor motility resulting in bacterial overgrowth), malabsorption (chronic pancreatitis), HIV/AIDS, or organ transplant.
- Social history: Secondary gain from diarrhea, alcohol use (chronic pancreatitis, bacterial overgrowth), sexual history, and HIV/AIDS risk factors.

- Family history: IBD, celiac disease, pancreatitis, hyperthyroidism, colon polyps, cancer, multiple endocrine neoplasia (MEN) syndrome.

Physical Examination

- Vital Signs: Fever, tachycardia and hypotension.
- HENT (**h**ead, **e**ars, **n**ose, **t**hroat): Signs of dehydration, oral ulcers, pallor, icterus, thyromegaly, lymphadenopathy, skin, rash, hyperpigmentation.
- Musculoskeletal: Arthritis.
- Abdomen: Tenderness to palpation, masses, hepatosplenomegaly.
- Respiratory: Wheezing.
- Cardiovascular: Tricuspid regurgitation.
- Extremities: Edema.
- Rectal: Blood, anal fissures, skin tags.

Clinical Manifestations (Box 2-1)

Osmotic Diarrhea

- Osmotic diarrhea should be suspected in patients with diarrhea that stops with fasting and in patients with large, voluminous, greasy, floating, malodorous stool.

BOX 2-1 Major Causes of Chronic Diarrhea

Infectious Diarrhea
- *Cryptosporidium, Giardia, Entamoeba histolytica,* Whipple's disease

Osmotic Diarrhea/Malabsorptive Diarrhea
- Medications/diet: Sorbitol sugar, lactose intolerance, magnesium-containing compounds, e.g., antacids, lactulose
- Pancreatic insufficiency: Chronic pancreatitis, cystic fibrosis, status post Whipple resection
- Bile salt insufficiency: Bacterial overgrowth, short bowel syndrome after small bowel resection, Crohn's ileitis
- Mucosal abnormality: Celiac disease, tropical sprue, Whipple disease, protein-losing enteropathy, small bowel lymphoma

Secretory Diarrhea
- Diet/medications: Stimulant laxatives, caffeine, ethanol, digoxin, colchicine, cholinergic agents, adrenal insufficiency
- Neuroendocrine tumors: VIPoma, mastocytosis, carcinoid tumor, Zollinger–Ellison syndrome, medullary carcinoma of the thyroid
- Altered motility: Hyperthyroidism, post vagotomy, irritable bowel syndrome
- Neoplasia: Villous adenoma, adenocarcinoma, lymphoma

Inflammatory Diarrhea
- IBD, collagenous colitis, microscopic colitis, radiation enteritis, vasculitis

- Ingestion of osmotically active solutes results in the retention of water.
- Stool osmotic gap = 290 – 2(Na + K). An osmotic gap >125 mOsm/kg is suggestive of an osmotic diarrhea.
- Dietary osmotic agents should be excluded by a careful history.
- Positive Sudan III stain, a qualitative test for fecal fat, suggests fat malabsorption.
- 72-h stool collection is a quantitative test that is rarely necessary to demonstrate fat malabsorption (normal <7 g/day).
- Stool acid steatocrit is a spot test for quantitative estimation of fecal fat.
- Further testing for carbohydrate malabsorption, lactose intolerance, bacterial overgrowth, antibodies for celiac sprue, and laxative screen to detect laxative abuse should be performed if the previous tests are negative and an osmotic diarrhea is suspected.

SECRETORY DIARRHEA

- Secretory diarrhea is large-volume watery diarrhea that persists with fasting.
- There is a characteristic small osmotic gap <50 mOsm/kg.
- To determine the etiology of secretory diarrhea TSH (hyperthyroidism), VIPoma (vasoactive intestinal peptide–producing), gastrin (gastrinoma), 5-hydroxy indole acetic acid (carcinoid) should be checked.
- Irritable bowel syndrome should be suspected in patients with long duration of symptoms >1 year with the absence of nocturnal diarrhea and no significant weight loss, dehydration, or electrolyte abnormalities.

INFLAMMATORY DIARRHEA

- Should be suspected in patients when diarrhea is fecal occult blood positive and fecal leukocytes are present.
- Stool cultures are needed to exclude infectious causes of diarrhea.
- Stool should be tested for *C. difficile* toxin.

Diagnosis (Fig. 2-1)

- Blood tests:
  - Complete blood count
  - Complete metabolic panel
  - Prothrombin time (PT)/partial thromboplastin time (PTT)/ INR
  - TSH (thyroid-stimulating hormone)
  - Antigliadin, antitissue transglutaminase antibody
  - Iron, B_{12}, folate, vitamin D levels

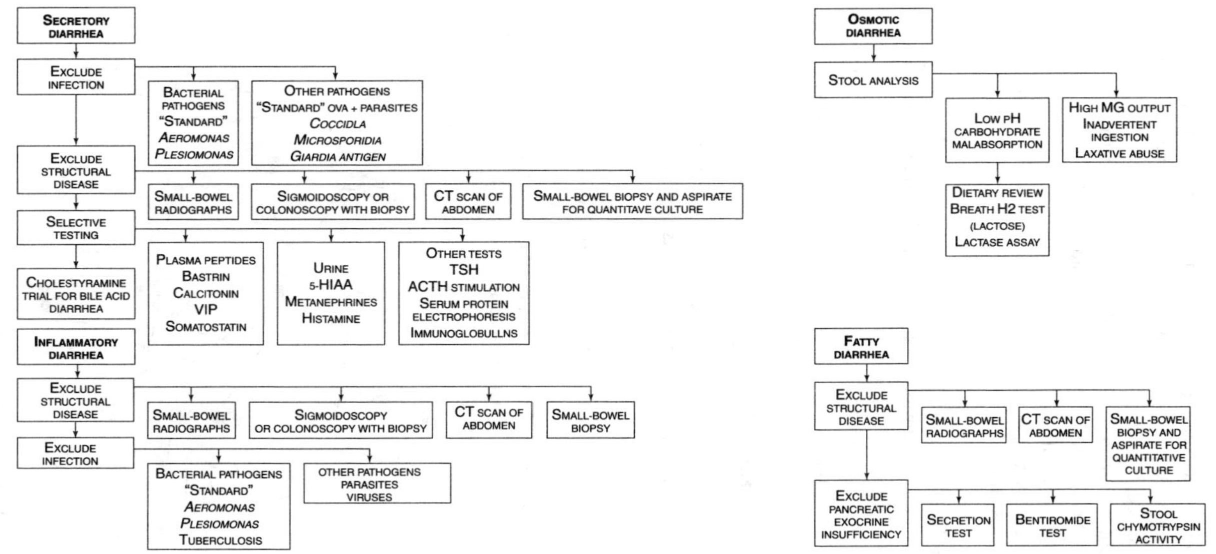

Figure 2-1 • Diagnostic approach to chronic diarrhea. (From Fine KD, Schiller LR. AGA technical review on the evaluation and management of chronic diarrhea. *Gastroenterology.* 1999;166:1464, with permission.)

- Stool tests:
  - Stool fecal leukocytes, although frequently performed, have a sensitivity of 70% and specificity of 50% for inflammatory diarrhea.
  - Fecal occult blood.
  - Stool electrolytes and osmolality for osmotic gap.
- The following tests should be considered:
  - *C. difficile* toxin
  - Stool ova and parasites
  - Stool cultures
  - Laxative screen
  - VIP, 5HIAA, gastrin, glucagon, calcitonin
- Endoscopic evaluation: Colonoscopy with biopsy, and in some cases EGD with biopsy to rule out sprue.
- Abdominal computed tomography (CT)/CT angiography may be needed in patients to rule out vascular insufficiency.

Acute Abdominal Pain

It is important to determine the etiology of acute abdominal pain in order to triage and to manage patients appropriately (Fig. 2-2)

History

The history may provide information that is pertinent to establishing a diagnosis:

- Onset: Sudden onset of abdominal pain that then becomes generalized suggests organ perforation.

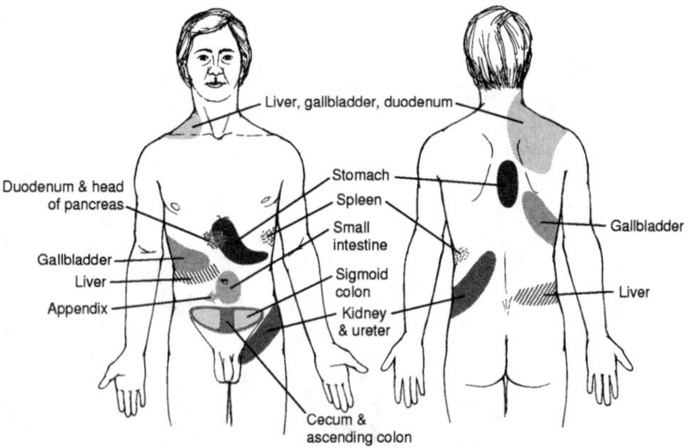

Figure 2-2 • Pain may be referred into the thoracic region from irritation of the internal organs in predictable patterns. (From Hendrickson T. *Massage for orthopedic conditions.* Philadelphia: Lippincott Williams & Wilkins; 2002, with permission.)

- Site of the pain: Visceral pain from organs derived from the embryonic foregut is epigastric, midgut in the periumbilical area, and hindgut in the hypogastrium.
- Intensity.
- Quality of pain: Pain from renal stones or from the colon is known as colic (intermittent and wringing).
- Radiation/progression: As the pain from the visceral organ begins to irritate somatic structures, pain is perceived in the area of the overlying muscle or skin with the same innervation as the visceral organ.
- Aggravating and relieving factors: Worsening with the even slight movement (movement of the bed/trip to the hospital) suggests peritoneal inflammation.
- Associated symptoms: Anorexia (often seen in patients with appendicitis), nausea, vomiting, diarrhea (ileitis or colitis), fever (infectious or inflammatory process), tenesmus, and urgency (colonic inflammation).
- Prior episodes: Peptic ulcer disease, pancreatitis, biliary colic, IBD, irritable bowel syndrome, chronic mesenteric ischemia are often sources of recurrent abdominal pain.
- Past history: Sickle cell disease, diabetes mellitus, diverticulosis, peptic ulcer disease, biliary colic, atrial fibrillation, hypertension, coronary artery disease, peripheral vascular disease, mesenteric ischemia, aortic aneurysm, HIV risk factors.
- Medications: NSAIDs, aspirin.
- Alcohol use: Gastritis, peptic ulcer disease, chronic pancreatitis should all be considered in patients with significant alcohol use.
- Recent travel and sick contacts: Infectious etiologies should be considered.
- Information on last menstrual period, vaginal discharge (pregnancy-related complications, fibroids, endometriosis, sexually transmitted diseases), past sexually transmitted diseases (tubo-ovarian abscess), and history of prior ectopic pregnancies (recurrent ectopic) should be sought.

Physical Examination

- Vital signs: Fever, tachycardia, and hypotension are signs of a serious systemic illness.
- Inspection:
  - Abdominal distension can be caused by fluid, fat, feces, flatulence, and fetus.
  - Visible scars from prior surgery should be noted as adhesions following surgery are a frequent cause of obstruction.
  - Peristaltic waves may be seen in cases of bowel obstruction.
  - Discoloration around the umbilicus (Cullen sign) or flank (Grey Turner sign) is seen in cases of splenic rupture and hemorrhagic pancreatitis due to retroperitoneal blood.

- Visible veins are seen in patients with cirrhosis with collateral veins radiating away from the umbilicus; in IVC obstruction, tortuous epigastric veins may be seen with blood flowing upward in the lower abdomen instead of in a downward direction to the groin.
- Hernia sites should be inspected to look for epigastric, umbilical, femoral, and inguinal hernias that may be incarcerated or strangulated.

- Palpation:
  - Localize the site of the pain.
  - Assess for guarding (voluntary contraction of the abdominal musculature in response to palpation; guarding can be overcome by asking patients to flex their knees), rigidity, and rebound tenderness (pain due to displacement of a deep-seated organ resulting in peritoneal irritation with the release of applied pressure on the abdomen). These signs may present late in cases of pelvic peritonitis and are best elicited by rectal examination.
  - It is important to differentiate intra-abdominal pain from abdominal wall pain. If contracting the rectus abdominis results in an increase in pain, the pain is likely to originate from the abdominal wall, whereas visceral pain decreases with contraction (Carnett sign).
- Percussion: Useful in the evaluation of ascites with shifting dullness and fluid thrill.
- Auscultation:
  - Absent bowel sounds suggest peritonitis or paralytic ileus. It is important to listen for 3 min before deciding they are absent.
  - Increased frequency or intensity of bowel sounds suggests a small bowel obstruction or intestinal obstruction (tinkling quality); in carcinoid syndrome, patients have characteristically loud borborygmi.
- Rectal and pelvic exam.

Acute Appendicitis

Acute appendicitis occurs secondary to obstruction of the appendiceal lumen from a fecalith, appendiceal calculus, or lymphoid hyperplasia.

Clinical Manifestations

Presents with acute onset of abdominal pain that is poorly localized to the periumbilical area (visceral pain) and then to the right lower quadrant (McBurney point between the umbilicus and anterior superior iliac spine) as the parietal peritoneum comes into contact with the inflamed appendix.

- Associated nausea, vomiting, anorexia.
- Low-grade fever.
- Patients with pelvic appendix exhibit atypical symptoms
- High-grade fever and the presence of an abdominal mass signify perforation of the appendix and development of a phlegmon or abscess.

Physical Examination

- McBurney point tenderness (McBurney point lies at the junction of the lateral one third and the medial two thirds of the line joining the right anterior superior iliac spine to the umbilicus).
- Obturator sign: Pain on external rotation of the flexed thigh.
- Psoas sign: Pain on extension of the right thigh.

Diagnosis

- Blood tests: Mild leukocytosis is frequently seen.
- Abdominal CT: Highly sensitive and specific and helps to differentiate acute appendicitis from other causes of abdominal pain.
- Pelvic ultrasound: To rule out a pelvic pathology in women with abdominal pain.

Differential Diagnosis

Mesenteric adenitis, cecal diverticulitis, Meckel diverticulitis, and pelvic inflammatory disease.

Treatment

- Appendectomy is indicated in patients with uncomplicated appendicitis.
- Appendiceal rupture and abscess can be managed conservatively with antibiotics and CT-guided drainage.

Perforated Duodenal Ulcer

Clinical Manifestations

- Presents with sudden onset of severe epigastric pain followed by diffuse abdominal pain in elderly individuals.
- Pain is aggravated by movement and respiration. Patients therefore try to remain perfectly still.
- Subphrenic collection of gastric contents may cause radiation of pain to the scapula.
- Low-grade fever and tachycardia are often present.

Diagnosis

- Upright films of the abdomen demonstrate air under the diaphragm.
- Abdominal CT with water-soluble contrast is used to confirm the diagnosis and the site of perforation.

Treatment

- Operative closure of the perforation, peritoneal debridement, and definitive surgery for ulcers is the treatment of choice.
- In unstable patients, omental closure with *H. pylori* treatment may be performed.

Abdominal Aortic Aneurysm

These are usually asymptomatic until rupture occurs. Expansion of an aneurysm results in mild abdominal or back pain, but it is when it ruptures that it presents with the acute onset of severe abdominal pain, pulsatile mass in the abdomen, and hypotension from hemorrhage. Abdominal aortic aneurysm may rupture and be temporarily contained, but if the diagnosis is suspected further management needs to be operative (Box 2-2).

BOX 2-2 Causes of Acute Abdominal Pain by Location

Epigastric Pain
- Gastritis
- Peptic ulcer
- Pancreatitis
- Angina

Right Upper Quadrant
- Acute cholecystitis
- Acute cholangitis
- Choledocholithiasis
- Nephrolithiasis

Left Upper Quadrant
- Splenomegaly
- Splenic infarction
- Splenic rupture
- Nephrolithiasis

Right Lower Quadrant Pain
- Appendicitis
- Cecal diverticulitis
- Meckel diverticulitis
- Mesenteric adenitis
- Crohn's ileitis
- Amoeboma
- Ileocecal tuberculosis
- Ovarian torsion
- Tubo-ovarian abscess
- Ruptured ectopic
- Uterine leiomyoma

Left Lower Quadrant Pain
- Diverticulitis
- Nephrolithiasis
- Ovarian torsion
- Tubo-ovarian abscess
- Ruptured ectopic
- Uterine leiomyoma

Suprapubic (Hypogastric) Pain
- Bladder distension
- Acute cystitis

BOX 2-3 Lists Other Causes of Abdominal Pain that Should be Considered

Mesenteric ischemia: Pain is most often periumbilical, but the site depends on the vascular territory.
Appendagitis epiploica: Inflammation of the peritoneal fat containing appendages secondary to torsion or spontaneous thrombosis of the draining vein can present with acute onset of abdominal pain.
Familial Mediterranean fever: Patients have recurrent attacks of abdominal pain and fever and other signs of serositis that resolve spontaneously.
Rectus sheath hematoma: Pain is localized to a well-defined area and pain increases with contraction of the anterior abdominal wall, whereas visceral pain decreases with contraction (Carnett sign).
Lower lobe pneumonia
Herpes zoster
Diabetic ketoacidosis
Sickle crisis due to vaso-occlusion

Other Causes of Abdominal Pain

Box 2-3 lists other causes of abdominal pain that should be considered.

Chapter

3 Diseases of the Esophagus

Gastroesophageal Reflux Disease

Epidemiology

- Gastroesophageal reflux disease (GERD) is one of the most prevalent gastrointestinal disorders.
- Of individuals with GERD, 10% to 15% have heartburn or regurgitation at least once a week and 5% to 9% have symptoms every day.
- Symptoms of GERD are secondary to the backflow of gastric contents into the esophagus.

Etiology/Pathogenesis

- Decreased lower esophageal sphincter (LES) tone.
- Transient relaxation of the LES.
- Secondary causes of LES incompetence:
  - Scleroderma-like diseases
  - Increased intra-abdominal pressure: Pregnancy, ascites, tight clothes, and obesity
  - Dietary factors: Caffeine, nicotine, and peppermint
  - Medications: Anticholinergic drugs, beta-agonists, aminophylline, nitrates, calcium channel blockers

Clinical Manifestations

- The majority of patients are asymptomatic.
- Regurgitation of gastric contents resulting in sour taste in the mouth and water brash.
- Retrosternal burning pain that is often confused with angina.
- Reflux into the pharynx and larynx can result in pharyngitis, laryngitis, with resultant cough and hoarseness of voice. Nocturnal worsening of cough and a chronic cough for >3 weeks is highly suggestive of GERD.
- Recurrent pulmonary aspiration can cause aspiration pneumonia, as well as bronchospasm. GERD should be considered in patients with nocturnal cough and wheezing.
- Persistent dysphagia can result from the development of a peptic stricture.

- Rapidly progressive dysphagia and weight loss may be seen with adenocarcinoma in an area of Barrett's esophagus.
- Hematemesis from esophagitis or ulceration.

Diagnosis

The diagnosis of GERD is a clinical one, and patients are treated with an empiric course of antireflux medication. Diagnostic studies are indicated in patients with persistent symptoms, those who do not respond to therapy, and those who have developed complications of GERD.

- Barium swallow is usually normal in uncomplicated esophagitis but may reveal a stricture or ulceration due to GERD.
- Upper endoscopy may reveal the presence of erosive esophagitis, ulceration, peptic stricture, Barrett's esophagus (intestinal metaplasia of the lower esophagus replacing the normal squamous epithelium with columnar epithelium), or adenocarcinoma. However, the endoscopic appearance may be normal in non-erosive esophagitis, and biopsy provides a definitive diagnosis.
- Use of a 24-h pH probe is necessary only when the diagnosis of reflux is unclear, particularly in the evaluation of chest pain without endoscopic features of esophagitis.
- Bernstein test involves the infusion of hydrochloric acid or normal saline into the esophagus. In patients with symptomatic esophagitis, infusion of acid (not of saline) reproduces the symptoms of reflux. However, reproduction of pain on infusion of acid does not necessarily correlate with periods of reflux and acidity of the esophagus seen on 24-h pH monitoring.
- Esophageal motility study confirms the incompetence of the LES. It is necessary prior to surgical repair of the esophagus to determine esophageal motor function abnormalities.

Differential Diagnosis

Angina, peptic ulcer disease, and esophageal dysmotility.

Treatment

- Lifestyle modification
  - Weight loss.
  - Elevation of the head end of the bed by about 4 to 6 in.
  - Smoking cessation.
  - Dietary modification to avoid the consumption of fatty foods, coffee, chocolate, alcohol, mint, and orange juice.
  - Discontinuation of medications associated with reflux.
- Acid suppression and treatment of complications:
  - H2 receptor blockers are useful in mild cases of GERD.
  - Proton pump inhibitors (PPI) are more effective in healing erosive esophagitis.

- Neutralization of bile with cholestyramine or sucralfate is useful in alkaline esophagitis.
- Esophagogastroduodenoscopy (EGD) should be performed in patients suspected of complications such as bleeding, stricture, and in patients with longstanding reflux to rule out the development of Barrett's esophagus.
- Peptic strictures are treated with endoscopic dilatation.
- There are limited data to support the role of *Helicobacter pylori* in GERD and, currently, testing for *H. pylori* in patients with GERD is not the standard of care.

• Antireflux surgery
  - Surgery is indicated in individuals who develop complications of GERD such as bleeding, ulceration, stricture, Barrett's esophagus, or who cannot tolerate PPI therapy. Motility studies are essential prior to surgery.
  - Nissen fundoplication involves wrapping the gastric fundus around the esophagus, which increases the LES pressure.

Complications

• Reflux esophagitis
• Peptic stricture results from resultant fibrosis in the distal esophagus
• Barrett's esophagus is intestinal metaplasia of the normal esophageal squamous epithelium
• Adenocarcinoma of the distal esophagus in areas of Barrett's esophagus.

Barrett's Esophagus

Etiology/Pathogenesis

• Barrett's esophagus is defined as the metaplasia of esophageal squamous epithelium by more resistant columnar epithelium secondary to longstanding reflux esophagitis.
• More common in white males, with an increase in prevalence with age.
• Barrett's epithelium becomes dysplastic and then progresses to adenocarcinoma at a rate of 0.5%/year.
• Barrett's esophagus is divided into long-segment (>2 to 3 cm) or short-segment (<2 to 3 cm).
• Long-segment Barrett's esophagus is seen in ~5% patients and short-segment Barrett's esophagus in up to 15% of patients who have undergone endoscopy for chronic GERD.
• Long-segment disease has a higher risk of dysplasia and adenocarcinoma than short-segment Barrett's esophagus.

Diagnosis

- All patients with persistent GERD symptoms at age 50 should undergo an EGD to identify areas of Barrett's epithelium.

Treatment

- Established metaplasia does not regress with treatment; therefore, acid suppression and fundoplication are indicated only when active esophagitis is also present.
- Surveillance frequency depends on the risk of developing esophageal adenocarcinoma and is therefore related to the length of involved esophageal mucosa.
- Short segments of Barrett's esophagus (distal 2 to 3 cm) appear to be at low risk and are not routinely surveyed.
- Patients with long-segment Barrett's esophagus are advised to have endoscopic surveillance at 1-year intervals for 2 years and then every 2 to 3 years. The frequency of surveillance is increased if dysplasia is detected.
- High-grade dysplasia is treated by esophagectomy of the Barrett's segment. Laser or thermocoagulative mucosal ablation and endoscopic mucosal resection (EMR) are being evaluated as alternatives.

ESOPHAGITIS

Infectious Esophagitis

- Herpes simplex virus 1 (HSV 1) and HSV 2 can cause esophagitis. Both are seen in immunocompromised individuals, whereas HSV 1 occurs in immunocompetent patients.
- Cytomegalovirus (CMV) esophagitis occurs in immunocompromised individuals, and ulcers are typically in the distal esophagus.
- Acute HIV may be associated with esophageal ulceration at the time of seroconversion.
- *Candida* esophagitis is also seen in immunodeficient states and patients may have concomitant oral candidiasis.

Clinical Manifestations

- Retrosternal chest pain that may be confused with angina.
- Dysphagia (difficulty swallowing) and odynophagia (pain on swallowing).
- Systemic symptoms with fevers, chills, nausea, and vomiting may be seen.
- Herpetic vesicles or oral thrush may be seen.
- Rarely, esophagitis is associated with esophageal perforation and fistula formation.

Diagnosis

- EGD with biopsy and culture is needed to make a definitive diagnosis. However, in immunocompromised patients with suspected esophageal candidiasis, empiric treatment should be initiated. Patients who fail to respond can then undergo an EGD to make a definitive diagnosis.

Treatment

- Nystatin oral suspension for oral thrush. Empiric therapy with fluconazole for 1 week for esophageal candidiasis. Patients who are unable to tolerate oral medication are treated with intravenous fluconazole or amphotericin B.
- HSV esophagitis is treated with antiviral such as acyclovir orally. Intravenous acyclovir is reserved for severe cases, and treatment is with foscarnet in cases of acyclovir resistance.
- CMV esophagitis is treated with 2 to 4 weeks of gancyclovir given intravenously or with oral valgancyclovir. Resistant cases are treated with foscarnet.

Radiation Esophagitis

- Radiation esophagitis is seen in patients receiving external beam radiation therapy for a thoracic malignancy and is often the dose-limiting toxicity in these patients. Radiation esophagitis frequently results in stricture formation.
- Indomethacin may prevent radiation-induced damage and treatment is with viscous lidocaine for pain control.

Eosinophilic Esophagitis

Epidemiology/Pathogenesis

- Eosinophilic esophagitis affects adults 20 to 30 years old; men are affected more often than women. Among children, boys are affected more than girls.
- Patients often have a history of allergies and of food impaction due to underlying dysmotility.

Clinical Manifestations

- Eosinophilic esophagitis mimics gastroesophageal reflux disease and often causes solid food dysphagia.
- Esophagitis results in narrowing and stricture of the esophagus.
- Esophageal dysmotility may be seen with involvement of the muscular layer and food impaction may occur.

- Eosinophilic esophagitis should be suspected in patients with a history of allergies who present with GERD and fail to respond to acid suppression.

Diagnosis

- Laboratory tests: Eosinophilia and elevated immunoglobulin E (IgE) levels.
- EGD with biopsy shows mucosal eosinophilia.

Treatment

- Clinical and histologic improvement with diet elimination therapy.
- Inhaled or oral steroids.
- Acid suppression in cases with associated reflux.

Pill Esophagitis

- Pill esophagitis results from prolonged contact of medications with the esophageal mucosa resulting in esophagitis in addition to the production of an acidic pH by culprit medications.
- Medications, such as bisphosphonates, quinidine, potassium, tetracycline derivatives, aspirin and other NSAIDs, can cause esophagitis or discrete ulcers.
- Prevention involves taking such medications with large quantities of liquid while sitting upright for 1/2 h following administration of the medication.

Corrosive Esophagitis

Epidemiology/Pathogenesis

- Corrosive esophagitis results from ingestion of acid or alkaline substances.
- Acid ingestion results in superficial coagulation necrosis and eschar formation that protects the underlying layers of the esophagus.
- Alkaline burns result in liquefaction necrosis of all the layers of the esophagus and can result in perforation, mediastinitis, and death.
- Box 3-1 presents a grading system for esophageal burns.

Clinical Manifestations

- Retrosternal burning pain.
- Excess salivation and drooling due to the inability to swallow secretions.
- Gagging secondary to esophageal spasm.
- Persistent abdominal pain with guarding, rigidity, and rebound suggests esophageal or gastric perforation.

BOX 3-1 Grading System for Esophageal Burns to Predict Clinical Outcomes

Grade 0: Normal mucosa
Grade 1: Mucosal edema and hyperemia
Grade 2A: Superficial ulcers, bleeding, or exudates
Grade 2B: Deep discrete focal or circumferential ulcers
Grade 3A: Multiple ulcers with focal necrosis
Grade 3B: Multiple ulcers with extensive necrosis

Zagar SA et al. The role of fiberoptic endoscopy in the management of corrosive ingestion and modified classification of burns. *Gastrointestinal endoscopy* 37(2):165–169, 1991.

- Severe retrosternal or back pain is suggestive of esophageal perforation and mediastinitis.
- Hoarseness and stridor may be seen with burns of the pharynx and larynx.
- Pulmonary aspiration may result in pneumonia.

Treatment

- Symptomatic patients should be carefully monitored with the aim to identify complications such as perforation, peritonitis mediastinitis, and acute respiratory distress syndrome with serial chest radiography and abdominal films.
- Nil per oral (NPO).
- Intravenous fluids and correction of electrolyte abnormalities.
- Pain control with intravenous medications.
- Neutralization of acid/alkali, use of a nasogastric tube, and the induction of emesis are all contraindicated due to an increased risk of perforation.
- There is no role for steroids or antibiotics in corrosive esophagitis.
- EGD should be performed within 24 to 48 h of injury to assess the degree of mucosal damage, guide management, and provide prognostic information.
- Severe cases may need esophagogastrectomy with colon interposition.

Complications

- Stricture formation: 70% to 100% of patients with grade 2B and 3 injury develop stricture formation with resultant dysphagia. This may occur between 2 months and several years after the ingestion.
- Squamous cell carcinoma: The risk is up to 1,000 times higher compared to the general population, and therefore surveillance endoscopy is recommended for 15 to 20 years following ingestion at 1-year to 3-year intervals.

ESOPHAGEAL MOTILITY DISORDERS

Achalasia (Fig. 3-1)

Epidemiology/Pathogenesis

- Achalasia, a major motor disorder of the esophagus, is characterized by impaired swallow-induced relaxation of the smooth muscle of the lower esophageal sphincter and the absence of esophageal peristalsis.
- The region of the LES shows degeneration of the myenteric plexus and a marked reduction in nitric oxide synthase.
- Achalasia most commonly affects individuals between 30 and 60 years old, but can occur in any age group.

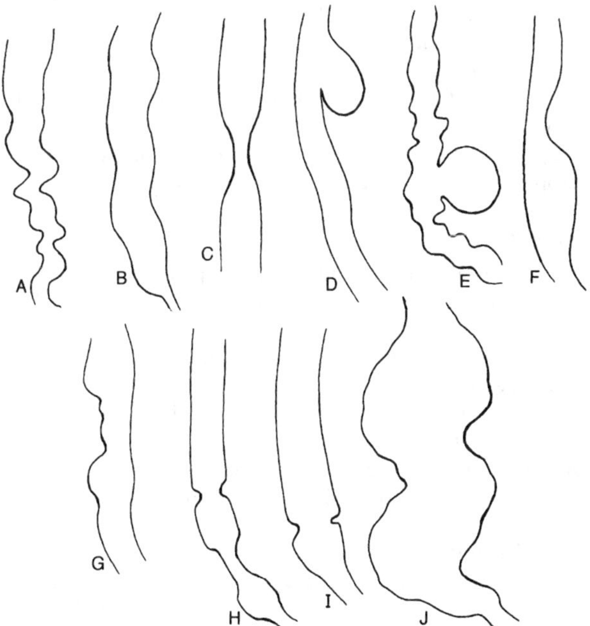

Figure 3-1 • Various barium studies. **A:** Diffuse spasm; **B:** achalasia (moderate); **C:** carcinoma, annular type; **D:** Zenker's diverticulum; **E:** diffuse spasm with epiphrenic diverticulum; **F:** leiomyoma; **G:** carcinoma, fungating type; **H:** sliding hiatus hernia (type I) with Barrett's esophagus and esophageal stricture due to reflux; **I:** Schatzki ring; **J:** achalasia (severe). (From Blackbourne LH. *Advanced surgical recall*, 2nd ed. Baltimore: Lippincott Williams & Wilkins; 2004, with permission.)

Clinical Manifestations

- Dysphagia to both solids and liquids is classic of a motility disorder.
- Regurgitation of contents of the esophagus is frequently seen.
- Chest pain.
- Heartburn from irritation of the lining of the esophagus by food.
- Weight loss that may be significant in some cases.
- Globus, a sensation of a lump in the throat, may be the presenting feature.
- An incidental finding on chest radiograph may show a widened mediastinum secondary to esophageal dilatation and the absence of the gastric air bubble due to the failure of the LES to relax.

Diagnosis

- Barium esophagram shows a characteristic "bird beak" appearance with tapering of the large dilated esophagus to a small narrowed segment due to a contracted LES.
- Esophageal manometry demonstrates an elevated resting LES pressure, incomplete relaxation in response to swallow, and lack of peristalsis of the smooth muscle in the body of the esophagus.
- Upper endoscopy is necessary to exclude malignancies at the esophagogastric junction that can mimic achalasia.

Treatment

- The aperistalsis in the body of the esophagus is usually irreversible, but peristalsis may be partially restored if the sphincter pressure is reduced.
- Nitrates and calcium-channel blockers taken before meals have limited efficacy.
- Pneumatic dilation of the lower esophageal sphincter.
- Surgical myotomy.
- *Botulinum* toxin decreases LES pressure by blocking the release of acetylcholine from the myenteric plexus.

Complications

- Esophageal ulceration, candidiasis, progression to malignancy.

Differential Diagnosis

- Cancer of the esophagogastric junction should be suspected in patients with advanced age >60 years, rapid weight loss, and difficulty in passing the endoscope through the gastroesophageal junction of a nondilated esophagus.
- Chaga disease and infiltrative diseases such as sarcoidosis and amyloidosis should also be considered.

Diffuse Esophageal Spasm

Epidemiology/Pathogenesis

Diffuse esophageal spasm (DES) is a motility disorder of the esophagus characterized by nonperistaltic contractions that are of large amplitude and duration. The disorder is secondary to decreased endogenous nitric oxide synthesis and/or degeneration of nerve processes.

Clinical Manifestations

- Retrosternal chest pain either at rest or after a swallow that lasts a few seconds to hours.
- Dysphagia to solids and liquids.

Diagnosis

- Barium swallow shows a characteristic "corkscrew" pattern due to simultaneous contraction of large areas of the esophagus.
- Esophageal manometry shows nonperistaltic contractions.

Treatment

- Calcium-channel blockers
- Nitrates

Complications

- DES can progress to achalasia.

Nutcracker Esophagus and Hypertensive Lower Esophageal Sphincter

Nutcracker esophagus is characterized by distal peristaltic high-amplitude contractions. Hypertensive LES is characterized by elevated resting pressure of the LES > 45 mm Hg. Clinical presentation is similar to DES, with retrosternal chest pain and dysphagia to solids and liquids. Confirm the diagnosis by barium swallow and manometry and treat with nitrates and calcium-channel blockers. Tricyclic antidepressants have also been shown in studies to decrease chest pain effectively in such disorders.

Scleroderma Esophagus

Epidemiology/Pathogenesis

- Scleroderma affects the mid and distal one third of the esophagus.
- Esophageal involvement is seen in patients with CREST (calcinosis, Raynaud's phenomenon, esophageal dysmotility, sclerodactyly, and telangiectasia) and progressive systemic sclerosis.

- Scleroderma esophagus is characterized by a decrease or absence of peristalsis secondary to smooth muscle atrophy and fibrosis and incompetence of the lower esophageal sphincter.

Clinical Manifestations

- Progressive dysphagia to solids and liquids.
- Decreased LES tone results in reflux of gastric contents (GERD) and symptoms of heartburn.
- Patients may have associated gastrointestinal manifestations of scleroderma, including delayed gastric emptying with resultant vomiting, gastric antral venous ectasia (GAVE) with upper GI bleeding, and iron-deficiency anemia. Decreased small bowel motility results in bacterial overgrowth and malabsorption, and altered large bowel motility results in constipation and fecal incontinence.

Diagnosis

- Barium swallow: Dilatation and decreased peristalsis of the mid-distal esophagus.
- Manometry: Decreased smooth muscle contraction and decreased LES resting pressure although the sphincter shows normal relaxation.

Treatment

- Treatment consists of treating GERD symptoms with H2 blockers or PPIs.

Hiatus Hernia

- Hiatus hernia is the herniation of the stomach through a diaphragmatic opening (Fig. 3-2).
- Type I: Sliding hiatal hernia is one in which the gastroesophageal junction and the fundus of the stomach are herniated upward.
- Type II: This is a pure paraesophageal hernia in which the gastroesophageal junction remains fixed and a pouch of the stomach herniates through the esophageal hiatus of the diaphragm.
- Type III: This hernia has elements of type I and II, with herniation of the fundus and displacement of the gastroesophageal junction above the diaphragm.
- Type IV: In type IV, there is a large defect in the phrenoesophageal membrane resulting in the herniation of other organs such as the small bowel, colon, pancreas, and spleen.

Clinical Manifestations

- Small sliding hernias are usually asymptomatic and are discovered incidentally.
- Reflux esophagitis with retrosternal burning pain.

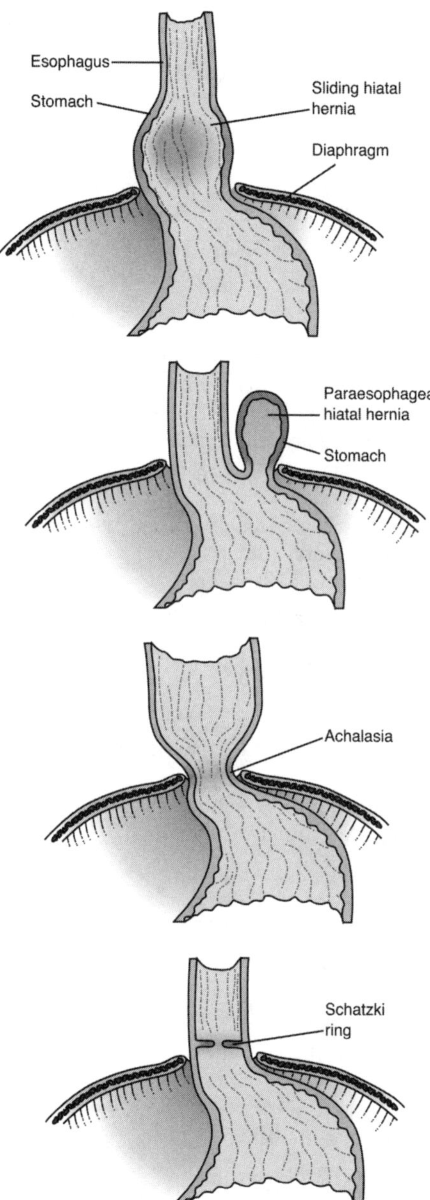

Figure 3-2 • Disorders of the esophageal outlet. (From Rubin E, Farber JL. *Pathology,* 3rd ed. Philadelphia: Lippincott Williams & Wilkins; 1999, with permission.)

- Intermittent bleeding from associated esophagitis, erosions (Cameron ulcers) leading to iron-deficiency anemia.
- Gastric volvulus or torsion may result in chest pain and dysphagia.

Diagnosis

- Barium swallow shows an outpouching of barium at the lower end of the esophagus, and free reflux of barium.
- EGD is used to diagnose complications such as erosive esophagitis, ulcers in the hiatal hernia, Barrett's esophagus, or malignancy.

Treatment

- Medical management with acid suppression with H2 blockers or PPIs for treatment of GERD.
- Surgery is indicated in patients with a sliding hiatus hernia who develop complications of GERD despite aggressive treatment with PPIs or in patients who do not want to continue antireflux medications, and in all cases of paraesophageal hernias because they do not regress and have a high rate of complications.
- Nissen fundoplication: This procedure involves a 360-degree fundic wrap around the gastroesophageal junction. The diaphragmatic hiatus is also repaired.
- Belsey (Mark IV) fundoplication: This operation involves a 270-degree wrap in an attempt to reduce the incidence of gas bloating and postoperative dysphagia. It is preferred when minimal esophageal dysmotility is suspected. To complete this operation, the left and right crura of the diaphragm are approximated.
- Hill repair: The cardia of the stomach is anchored to the posterior abdominal areas, such as the medial arcuate ligament. This also has the effect of augmenting the angle of His and thus strengthening the antireflux mechanism.

TUMORS OF THE ESOPHAGUS

Esophageal Cancer

Epidemiology/Pathogenesis

- Esophageal cancer, the seventh leading cause of cancer death in the United States, is predominately adenocarcinoma.
- Adenocarcinoma is more prevalent in whites and squamous cell cancer is more prevalent in blacks. Esophageal cancer is more prevalent in males, and patients are predominately older than 50 years.
- Approximately three quarters of all adenocarcinomas are found in the distal esophagus, whereas squamous cell carcinomas are more evenly distributed between the middle and lower third.

Risk Factors

- Smoking increases the risk of adenocarcinoma and squamous cell carcinoma.
- History of mediastinal radiation increases the risk of esophageal cancer
- Factors that increase risk of squamous cell cancer:
  - Alcohol consumption
  - Smoking
  - Achalasia
  - Radiation- or caustic-induced strictures
  - Plummer–Vinson syndrome/Patterson–Kelly syndrome
  - Tylosis, which is an autosomal dominant condition characterized by congenital hyperkeratosis of palms and soles
- Factors that increase risk of adenocarcinoma:
  - Barrett's esophagus, which can progress to develop adenocarcinoma
  - Cholecystectomy, which has been associated with adenocarcinoma due to reflux of bile in duodenal contents
  - Obesity
  - *Helicobacter pylori* may reduce the risk of severe GERD and be protective.

Clinical Manifestations

- Progressive dysphagia to solids and then liquids
- Odynophagia
- Significant weight loss (>10% in 6 months)
- Regurgitation of gastric contents, which can result in aspiration pneumonia
- Hoarseness of the voice due to involvement of the recurrent laryngeal nerve
- Chronic gastrointestinal blood loss with iron-deficiency anemia
- Tumor invasion of the aorta or pulmonary vessels, which are rare but may result in massive upper GI bleeding
- Tracheoesophageal fistula, a late complication of esophageal cancer
- Hypercalcemia, a paraneoplastic phenomenon associated with squamous cell carcinoma

Diagnosis

- EGD with cytologic brushing and biopsy is needed to make a definitive diagnosis.
- Endoscopic ultrasound (EUS) predicts the depth of tumor invasion and the extent of lymph-node involvement.
- Computed tomography (CT) scan of the chest and abdomen is used to determine the extent of tumor and metastatic disease.
- Positron emission tomography (PET) with fludeoxyglucose can identify metastatic disease that may be undetected by CT scan.

Treatment

- Esophageal cancer has poor prognosis with a less than 5% 5-year survival.
- Treatment of surgically respectable disease with preoperative chemotherapy and radiotherapy followed by surgical resection appears to prolong survival in a few randomized trials.
- Treatment of unresectable disease involves endoscopic dilation, esophageal stent placement, gastrostomy or jejunostomy for feeding, or endoscopic laser fulguration.

MISCELLANEOUS DISORDERS OF THE ESOPHAGUS

Lower Esophageal Ring (Schatzki Ring) (Fig. 3-2)

Epidemiology/Pathogenesis

- Consists of connective tissue with muscularis mucosa covered by squamous epithelium above and columnar epithelium below.
- Schatzki ring is almost always located close to the gastroesophageal junction.
- The pathogenesis of Schatzki ring is unclear, and chronic gastric reflux has been associated with mucosal rings.

Clinical Manifestations

- Lower esophageal rings are associated with intermittent solid food dysphagia.
- Unlike malignant strictures there is no associated weight loss.

Diagnosis

- Barium pill stops at the site of the ring.
- Endoscopy is less sensitive in detecting esophageal rings.

Treatment

- Endoscopic dilation
- Acid suppression therapy in patients with evidence of reflux or recurrent rings

Esophageal Web (Plummer–Vinson Syndrome/Kelly–Patterson Syndrome)

Epidemiology/Pathogenesis

- Usually located in the upper esophagus.
- More often seen in women and is classically associated with iron-deficiency anemia.
- Often a manifestation of systemic disease such as pemphigus vulgaris, epidermolysis bullosa, or bullous pemphigoid.

Clinical Manifestations

- Intermittent dysphagia to solids
- Iron-deficiency anemia with angular stomatitis, glossitis, and koilonychia

Treatment

- Iron supplementation
- Endoscopic balloon dilation

Differential Diagnosis

- Eosinophilic esophagitis

Esophageal Diverticulum

Esophageal diverticulae are outpouchings of the esophageal wall and are divided into three based on the layers involved.

- True diverticulum: Contains all the layers of the wall
- False diverticulum: Contains only the mucosa and submucosa
- Intramural diverticulum: Contains only the submucosa

Zenker's Diverticulum

Zenker's diverticulum is a false diverticulum that results from an outpouching of the esophageal mucosa posteriorly between the cricopharyngeus muscle and the inferior pharyngeal constrictor muscles.

Epidemiology/Pathogenesis

The etiology is incompletely understood and may be secondary to improperly timed relaxation of the cricopharyngeus muscle during swallowing. With longstanding increased pressure, the esophageal mucosa herniates posteriorly creating a false diverticulum.

Clinical Manifestations

Zenker's diverticulum frequently results in the retention of food and medication within it and leads to the following symptoms:

- Halitosis
- Dysphagia
- Regurgitation of food into the mouth
- Aspiration of retained food
- Visible mass in the neck
- Ulceration and bleeding secondary to retained medications

Diagnosis

- Barium swallow is diagnostic (Fig. 3-1).
- Endoscopy is indicated if the contrast study shows esophageal mucosal irregularities suggestive of neoplasia.

- Esophageal manometry is indicated if achalasia or another esophageal motility disorder is suspected from the barium swallow.

Treatment

- Small, asymptomatic diverticula require no specific therapy.
- For all others, surgical treatment consists of division of the cricopharyngeus muscle with or without diverticulectomy.
- Midesophageal diverticulum may be secondary to traction or adhesions. Epiphrenic diverticula may be associated with achalasia. Diverticula associated with motor abnormalities are treated with distal myotomy.

Mallory–Weiss Tear

Epidemiology/Pathogenesis

Mallory–Weiss tear is a longitudinal mucosal laceration at the gastroesophageal junction or gastric cardia caused by repeated retching. Patients are predominantly men between 40 and 50 years of age and often have a history of associated alcohol use.

Clinical Manifestations

- The classic presentation consists of an episode of hematemesis following a bout of retching, vomiting, or vigorous coughing.
- Less common presenting symptoms include melena, hematochezia, syncope, and abdominal pain.

Diagnosis

- Barium or gastrografin studies should not be performed due to their low diagnostic sensitivity and because they limit endoscopic evaluation and therapy.

Treatment

- Endoscopy is the procedure of choice for both diagnosis and treatment.
- Most bleeding stops spontaneously. Continued bleeding may respond to vasopressin or angiographic embolization.
- Surgery is indicated in rare cases.

Chapter 4

Diseases of the Stomach and Small Intestine

Peptic Ulcer Disease

An ulcer is characterized by loss of the surface epithelium >5 mm, that extends up to or penetrates the muscularis mucosa. Peptic ulcers usually occur in the stomach and duodenum but can occur in the esophagus, small bowel, at gastroenteric anastomoses, and in areas of ectopic gastric mucosa.

Epidemiology/Pathogenesis

The estimated lifetime prevalence of peptic ulcer disease is approximately 11% to 14% in men and 8% to 11% in women. Genetic predisposition, diet, and stress have not been conclusively proved to be causative. Factors implicated in the pathogenesis of peptic ulcers are as follows:

- *Helicobacter pylori:* The exact mechanism by which *H. pylori* causes ulcers is not known, but the following mechanisms have been proposed.
  - Urease produced by *H. pylori* allows the organisms to live in the acidic gastric environment and generate ammonia, which damages epithelial cells.
  - Lipopolysaccharide antigens cross-react with epithelial antigens resulting in gastritis.
  - Gastric metaplasia of the duodenum permits *H. pylori* to bind to it and results in further injury.
  - Increased gastric acid production secondary to an increase in gastrin or decrease in somatostatin.
  - Decreased bicarbonate production.
- Nonsteroidal antiinflammatory drugs (NSAIDs):
  - NSAIDs are responsible for dyspepsia, ulceration, and perforation in ~1.5% of users per year.
  - Risk factors for NSAID-induced ulcers are increasing dose of NSAIDs, concomitant steroid or anticoagulants use, *H. pylori* infection, smoking, alcohol use, and increasing age.
  - NSAID-induced ulcers are secondary to prostaglandin inhibition that results in decreased epithelial cell turnover; increased acid production; decreased mucosal bicarbonate, mucin and phospholipids production; and direct toxicity.
- Cigarette smoking: Does not increase acid production but may be associated with decreased mucosal blood flow, decreased

prostaglandin, direct free radical injury, and may increase the risk of *H. pylori* infections.

- Gastric hypersecretory states: Zollinger–Ellison syndrome should be considered if a patient has multiple ulcers, ulcers in areas other than the stomach and duodenum, or recurrent ulcers.

Clinical Manifestations

- Epigastric abdominal pain is the most frequent symptom but is nonspecific.
- Classically, duodenal ulcer pain classically occurs 1 to 3 h after a meal and is relieved by food and antacids, whereas gastric ulcer pain is usually precipitated by food. However, these features are not always seen, and both ulcers can present with pain after eating.
- Patients may be asymptomatic and may present with anemia or complications such as perforation and hemorrhage.
- Associated nausea, vomiting, and weight loss may be seen with gastric ulcers but significant weight loss (>10% in 6 months) is suggestive of a gastric malignancy.

Physical Examination

- Succussion splash from gastric outlet obstruction due to edema or stricture formation.
- Tachycardia and hypotension are seen with significant blood loss.
- Guarding, rigidity, and rebound tenderness are suggestive of a perforation.

Diagnosis

Empiric treatment with acid-blocking agents can be instituted without further workup in patients <45 years old without weight loss, anemia, or signs of occult bleeding or vomiting.

- Endoscopy: Most sensitive and specific method of evaluating the GI tract and allows for biopsies to be taken to exclude malignancy.
- Barium swallow: Barium swallow has lower sensitivity than endoscopy. Further, it does not obviate the need for endoscopy and biopsy if there is evidence of gastric ulcers, which should always be biopsied due to their malignant potential. It is therefore not pursued if endoscopy is readily available. Duodenal ulcer is seen as a crater frequently in the duodenal bulb and gastric ulcers appear as craters with radiating gastric folds.
- Testing for *H. pylori:* This is an essential part of the evaluation for peptic ulcer disease.
- Serology: 80% sensitive, 90% specific, used to detect infection. Serology, however, remains positive even after eradication and is therefore not useful for follow-up.
- Urea breath test: 95% sensitive and specific, useful for follow-up after eradication.

- Stool antigen: >90% sensitive and specific, useful in confirming eradication; should be performed 4 to 6 weeks after eradication to avoid false-positive and false-negative results.
- Esophagogastroduodenoscopy (EGD) with rapid urease test: >90% sensitive and specific. False negative with the recent use of proton pump inhibitors (PPIs), antibiotics, bismuth products, or recent or active bleeding. It should always be performed if the patient is undergoing EGD to rule to malignancy.
- EGD with histology: Indicated if the urease test on biopsy is negative.

Differential Diagnosis

Nonulcer dyspepsia, Crohn's disease, pancreatitis, cholelithiasis, chronic mesenteric ischemia.

Complications

Hemorrhage (15% to 25%), perforation (2% to 3%), gastric outlet obstruction (2% to 3%), penetration into the colon, pancreas, liver, and biliary tree.

Treatment

Acid Suppression

- Antacids
  - Not used as primary therapy for peptic ulcer disease.
  - Chronic calcium carbonate use results in milk alkali syndrome (hypercalcemia, renal failure, and alkalosis).
  - Magnesium hydroxide causes diarrhea and should be avoided in patients with renal failure as hypermagnesemia can occur.
  - Aluminum hydroxide produces constipation and can cause neurotoxicity with long-term use.
- H2 blockers
  - Act by inhibiting the histamine 2 (H2) receptor on the parietal cell and therefore inhibit acid secretion. Onset of action is within 1 to 3 h.
- Proton pump inhibitors
  - Irreversibly inhibit H-K ATPase and inhibit all phases of acid secretion. PPIs are most effective when the parietal cell is stimulated and there is maximal H-K ATPase in the parietal cell (after prolonged fasting). Inhibition of the parietal cell by an H2 blocker therefore results in a decrease in efficacy of PPIs.
  - PPIs have delayed onset of action (inhibition of two thirds of maximal acid production after 5 days of administration) and a long half-life of up to 18 h.
  - Patients who do not respond to H2 blockers and have refractory duodenal ulcers benefit from PPI therapy.

Cytoprotective Agents

- Sucralfate and bismuth subsalicylate
  - Act as barriers from acid and enhance mucosal repair, stimulate bicarbonate and mucin secretion, and bind growth factors such as epidermal growth factor, thereby increasing both defense and repair.
  - Sucralfate should be avoided in chronic renal failure due to aluminum toxicity.
- Prostaglandin analogues (e.g., misoprostol)
  - Used for the prevention of NSAID-induced ulcers.
  - Enhance mucosal defense by bicarbonate production, stimulate mucosal blood flow, and decrease cell turnover.
  - Major side effects are diarrhea and uterine contractions. Prostaglandin analogues are therefore contraindicated in pregnancy.

H. pylori Eradication

- In patients who test positive for *H. pylori*, triple therapy consisting of two antibiotics and a PPI for 10 to 14 days is the standard of care.
- Triple therapy with regimens that include amoxicillin, clarithromycin, and lasoprazole (>90% success rate).
- If testing for *H. pylori* remains positive, it is likely due to a resistant organism, and quadruple therapy should be used with amoxicillin, metronidazole, clarithromycin, and tetracycline.

EGD

- Indicated for patients with gastric ulcer to document healing in 8 weeks or with ulcer complications such as hemorrhage, perforation, and outlet obstruction.

Surgery

- Surgery is reserved for refractory cases of ulcers, gastric outlet obstruction, ulcer perforation, and massive bleeding (Figs. 4-1 and 4-2).

Zollinger–Ellison Syndrome

Zollinger–Ellison syndrome (ZES) is characterized by multiple and refractory peptic ulceration secondary to increased gastric acid production by a gastrin-producing tumor.

■ Epidemiology/Pathogenesis

- Tumors are usually located in the gastrinoma triangle and most commonly in the pancreas. (Gastrinoma triangle is bounded superiorly by the junction of the cystic with the common bile duct, inferiorly by the second and third part of the duodenum and medically by the neck of the pancreas.)

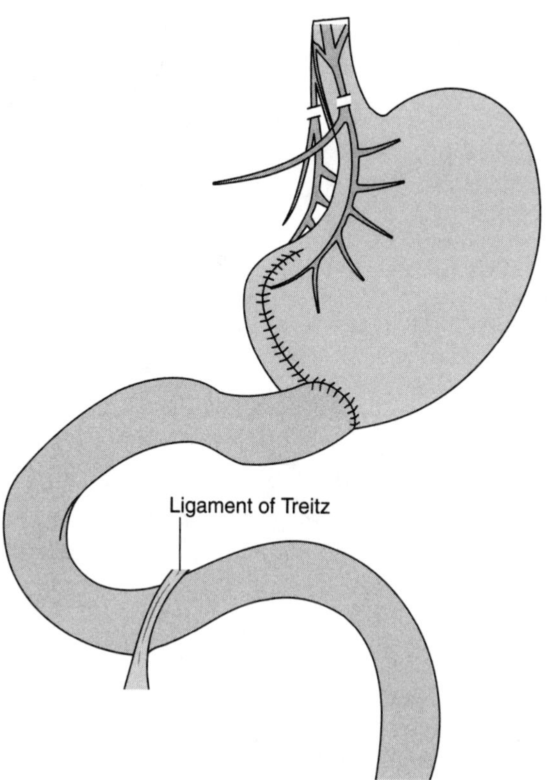

Figure 4-1 • Vagotomy and antrectomy with Billroth I anastomosis. (From Karp S, Morris J, Soybel, D. *Blueprints surgery.* 3rd ed. Oxford: Blackwell; 2004, with permission.)

- Gastrinomas are sporadic and less commonly familial. Multiple endocrine neoplasia (MEN 1), an autosomal dominant disorder (11 q11-q13) is characterized by tumors of the pituitary, pancreas, and parathyroid.

■ Clinical Manifestations

- Ulcers usually occur in the first part of the duodenum but a diagnosis of ZES should be considered if patients have the following features:
  - Ulceration in the second part of the duodenum and more distally
  - Multiple ulcers
  - Ulcers refractory to medical therapy or with frequent recurrence

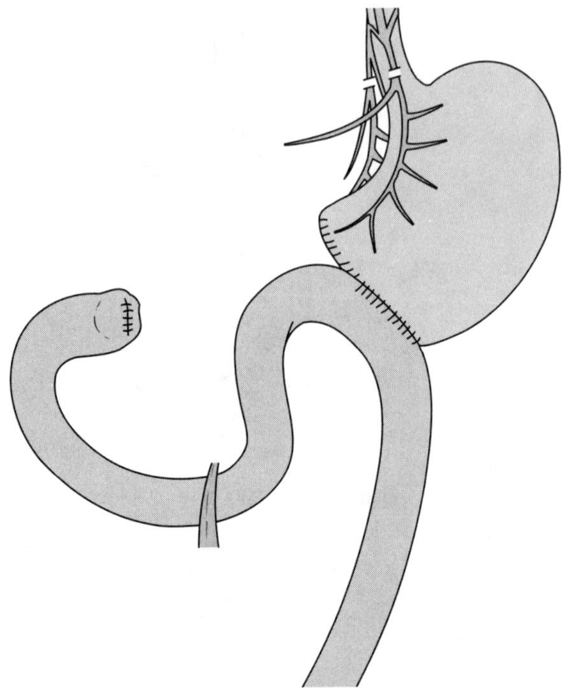

Figure 4-2 • Vagotomy and antrectomy with Billroth II anastomosis. (From Karp S, Morris J, Soybel, D. *Blueprints surgery*. 3rd ed. Oxford: Blackwell; 2004, with permission.)

- Ulcers with severe esophagitis
- Recurrence after surgery
- Ulceration in the absence of NSAID use or *H. pylori* infection
- Hypercalcemia
- Diarrhea of unknown etiology. Diarrhea in ZES is secondary to increased volume of gastric secretion, pancreatic enzyme inactivation by gastric acid resulting in malabsorption, damage to epithelial cells, and release of hormones such as vasoactive intestinal peptide (VIP)

Diagnosis

- Fasting gastrin level: Normal <150 pg/mL, gastrinoma gastrin level >150 to 200 pg/mL.
- Falsely elevated gastrin levels are seen in hypocholrhydria/achlorhydria, patients on PPI therapy, gastric outlet obstruction, renal insufficiency, and small bowel resection.

- Secretin stimulation test: Most sensitive and specific test for ZES. Based on the increase in gastrin to >200 pg/ml within 15 min of secretin administration.
- Tumor localization and staging: ^{111}In-pentreotide (octreoscan) with sensitivity and specificity >75% can be used to detect a gastrinoma. If lesions are detected in the liver, CT-directed liver biopsy can make the diagnosis. In the absence of metastatic disease, an EGD and endoscopic ultrasound (EUS) can be used to localize the tumor, but in cases where this is unrevealing selective angiography and portal vein sampling may be used.

Treatment

- PPIs are the treatment of choice.
- Somatostatin analogue octreotide has been found to be effective in decreasing tumor secretion and the growth of tumor metastases.
- Surgical resection of the gastrinoma is curative in patients without evidence of metastatic disease.
- In patients with metastatic disease, chemotherapy with streptozocin-containing regimens, interferon-alpha (IFN-α), and hepatic artery embolization have been used but have not been shown to improve mortality.

Prognosis

Depends on tumor size, location (duodenal wall better prognosis than pancreatic tumors), presence of metastatic disease, surgical resection (if complete, affords a near 100% survival rate and incomplete resection or unresectability carries a <50% 10-year survival), and gastrin levels (>10,000 pg/mL poor prognosis).

Nonulcer Dyspepsia

Nonulcer dyspepsia (NUD) is defined as chronic or recurrent upper abdominal pain or discomfort in the absence of an identifiable cause of organic disease after a diagnostic workup.

Epidemiology/Pathogenesis

- The causes of NUD are poorly understood.
- Several theories have been proposed including gastric hypersecretion, increased sensitivity to acid, exaggerated response to physiologic stimuli, abnormal motility, food intolerance, or a physical manifestation of a psychiatric pathology.

Classification

Classification of NUD is based on symptom subgroups. These subgroups do not correlate with the pathophysiology or response to therapy.

- Reflux-like (dyspepsia with heartburn or regurgitation)
- Ulcer-like
- Dysmotility-like

With the exception of "reflux-like dyspepsia," which is treated with PPI and is probably gastroesophageal reflux disease (GERD) and not NUD, these symptom subgroups are of little utility.

Clinical Manifestations

NUD cannot be reliably distinguished by history and physical examination from organic causes of dyspepsia.

- Vague abdominal discomfort.
- Bloating, belching, early satiety, nausea, occasional vomiting, and heartburn that are aggravated by meals.
- Nocturnal symptoms are uncommon.
- Symptoms tend to wax and wane and patients may be only minimally symptomatic in between.

Physical Examination

Patients with NUD characteristically have a normal physical exam.

Diagnosis

The diagnosis of NUD is a diagnosis of exclusion, and a detailed history that includes diet, medications, and life stresses should be sought.

- Laboratory studies: Complete blood count, electrolytes, calcium, TSH, erythrocyte sedimentation rate, and c-reactive protein are normal.
- Endoscopy: Patients with NUD have normal or nonspecific endoscopic findings. *Helicobacter pylori* testing in NUD is controversial.
- Abdominal imaging (CT abdomen): Should be considered for patients with longstanding symptoms if the above workup is negative and there is suspicion of a malignancy.

Treatment

- Trial of acid suppression with PPIs.
- Prokinetic agents such as metoclopramide have been shown to improve symptoms irrespective of the symptom profile.
- *H. pylori* eradication in patients who are positive.
- Antidepressants have been shown to benefit NUD due to a reduction in visceral sensitivity that is independent of their psychiatric effects.

Gastritis

Gastritis is inflammation of the mucosa secondary to injury, whereas in gastropathy there is epithelial damage without inflammation.

Classification (Rubin CE et al. *Gastroenterology*. 1997; 112:2108)

Diffuse Antral-Predominant Gastritis (DAG) with H. pylori

- The antrum is affected by *H. pylori* and diffuse inflammatory infiltrate is seen with a decrease in the number of glands.
- Duodenal and juxtapyloric ulcers may be present.
- DAG ulcers heal with *H. pylori* eradication.
- Risk of intestinal adenocarcioma is low.

Multifocal Atrophic Gastritis

- Multifocal intestinalized pangastritis (MIP) with or without *H. pylori*
  - MIP begins along the lesser curvature and extends proximally and distally
  - MIP can result in intestinal metaplasia (IM) that then becomes dysplasia and can progress to intestinal-type adenocarcinoma. Benign gastric ulcers that develop from IM regress with *H. pylori* eradication but IM does not.
- Nonulcer pangastritis (NUP) with *H. pylori*
  - NUP is infrequently associated with IM and rarely with gastric/duodenal ulcers and intestinal adenocarcinoma, IM. It regresses after eradication of *H. pylori*.

Diffuse Corporeal Atrophic Gastritis without H. pylori

- Confined to the gastric fundus.
  - Not associated with *H. pylori* but is associated with autoimmune disease.
- Destruction of the fundic glands results in atrophy and therefore achlorhydria and B_{12} malabsorption from loss of intrinsic factor.

Disorders of Absorption

Malabsorptive syndromes are characterized by steatorrhea or chronic watery diarrhea, increased flatus, weight loss, signs of vitamin and mineral deficiencies.

Clinical Manifestations

- Steatorrhea, consisting of the passage of pale, bulky, greasy stool that tends to float.
- Abdominal distention and flatus as result of fermentation of unabsorbed carbohydrates by colonic bacteria.
- Weight loss with severe panmalabsorption, but may not be seen in patients with more limited forms of malabsorption. If weight

loss is progressive, conditions such as inflammatory bowel disease (IBD) and malignancy should be considered.

- Anemia secondary to iron, folate or B_{12} deficiency with resultant glossitis, chelosis, and angular stomatitis.
- Deficiencies of the fat-soluble vitamins such as A, D, and K. Osteomalacia, bone pain, cramps, parasthesia, and tetany resulting from hypocalcemia. Vitamin K deficiency can cause easy bruising and ecchymosis, and vitamin A deficiency can produce night blindness.
- Constitutional symptoms of chronic fatigue and weakness.
- Associated dermatologic abnormalities; e.g., Whipple's disease is associated with hyperpigmentation, and dermatitis herpetiformis (pruritic, blistering skin eruption) is associated with celiac disease.

Diagnosis

Routine Blood Tests

- Complete blood count and serum chemistries: Anemia, hypokalemia, metabolic acidosis, hypocalcemia, and hypomagnesemia may be seen.
- Albumin levels are low; elevated PT and PTT suggest vitamin K malabsorption.
- Iron, folate, B_{12} levels, cholesterol, and triglyceride concentrations may be low.

Tests of Fat Absorption

- Sudan III stain: This is a simple and inexpensive test used to make a semiqunatitiative assessment of fat malabsorption. (Steatorrhea >5 droplets per high power field).
- 48-h or 72-h fecal fat: This test is the gold standard for determination of fat malabsorption but is rarely necessary and is an expensive test. Pancreatic exocrine insufficiency is associated with high stool fat concentrations (>10 g/100 g stool).

Tests of Carbohydrate Absorption

- Stool pH < 5.5 is classic for carbohydrate malabsorption secondary to bacterial fermentation but may not always be present.
- Osmotic Gap $= 290 - 2(\text{Na} + \text{K})$. Gap > 50 mOsm suggests osmotic diarrhea from carbohydrate malabsorption.
- D-xylose test whereby blood and urinary xylose concentration is measured fixed intervals after ingestion of 25 g of xylose. Failure of blood xylose levels to rise above 20 mg/100 mL at 1 h and above 22.5 mg/100 mL at 3 h or failure of urinary output to exceed 5 g/5 h suggests malabsorption from mucosal dysfunction because none of these sugars depends on pancreatic enzymes or bile acids for absorption. False-positive test:

Bacterial overgrowth in which substrate may be destroyed. Diabetes mellitus, dehydration, ascites, and impaired renal function also interfere with the test results.

- Hydrogen breath test: Simple, inexpensive test for malabsorption of a specific carbohydrate (e.g., due to disaccharidase deficiency). Rise of more than 10 to 20 ppm after ingestion of sucrose or lactose is consistent with malabsorption of the ingested substrate. False-positive tests occur in small bowel bacterial overgrowth. This produces an increase in breath hydrogen, but usually soon after ingestion. False-negative results can be seen in individuals in whom the colonic flora does not produce hydrogen and in patients on antibiotic therapy.

Measurement of Vitamin B_{12} Absorption

- Schilling test: Indicated in patients with suspected ileal disease.
- Radiolabeled B_{12} and exogenous intrinsic factor are given simultaneously by mouth, unlabeled B_{12} is given by injection to saturate internal B_{12} binding sites, and 24-h urinary recovery of the radiolabeled B_{12} is measured. Recovery of less than 9% of the administered dose is abnormal and suggests ileal dysfunction. False-positive results: Pancreatic exocrine insufficiency (because endogenous R-protein is normally cleaved by pancreatic enzymes from the R-protein–B_{12} complex), bacterial overgrowth, and renal failure.
- Dual-labeled Schilling test: Indicated to differentiate pancreatic insufficiency from bacterial overgrowth and ileal dysfunction. Two isotopes of cobalt are used to study the relative absorption of B_{12} coupled to R-protein and B_{12} coupled to intrinsic factor. Both complexes are labeled separately and given orally simultaneously. Urinary recovery of each isotope is measured. If pancreatic insufficiency is present, the B_{12} coupled with R-protein is malabsorbed and the ratio of isotopes in urine changes from the ratio that was administered. If bacterial overgrowth or ileal dysfunction is present, both B_{12} coupled to R-protein and B_{12} coupled to intrinsic factor are malabsorbed equally, and the ratio of the two isotopes is unchanged. Schilling test performed after the administration of antibiotics will be normal in patients with bacterial overgrowth but not in ileal dysfunction.

Evaluation of Bile Acid Malabsorption

- SeHCAT (selenium-75-labeled taurohomocholic acid) test: Radioactive taurocholic acid analogue is administered orally and total body retention is measured with repeat gamma scintigraphy over consecutive days. Retention of less than 50% after 3 days suggests bile acid malabsorption.

Tests for Small Bowel Bacterial Overgrowth

The principle behind the following tests is that bacterial metabolism of a substrate will release a measurable substance in exhaled air.

- ^{14}C xylose: Xylose in healthy individuals is absorbed from the small intestine and undergoes relatively slow metabolism when it reaches the colon. If bacteria are present in the upper GI tract or jejunum, xylose can be fermented and radioactive CO_2 will be exhaled in the breath within 60 min.
- Glucose-breath hydrogen test: A bolus of glucose is ingested and breath hydrogen concentrations are measured. If no bacteria are present in the upper GI tract or jejunum, the glucose is absorbed by the intestine and no hydrogen is generated. If bacteria are present, the glucose can be fermented before it can be absorbed and the hydrogen produced can be exhaled. The test has limited sensitivity as 20% people are colonized with bacteria that do not produce hydrogen.
- Quantitative culture of jejunal aspirate: The gold standard for bacterial overgrowth.

Tests for Pancreatic Function

- Bentiromide test: Detects severe pancreatic insufficiency. *N*-Benzoyl-*L*-tyrosyl-para-aminobenzoic acid is hydrolyzed by chymotrypsin and free para-aminobenzoic acid (PABA) is absorbed and excreted in the urine. False-positive results are seen in patients with severe mucosal disease, liver and renal insufficiency, and diabetes.

Celiac Sprue

Celiac sprue is characterized by malabsorption resulting from ingestion of gluten, with characteristic histologic appearance of villous flattening with lymphocytic infiltration; and both clinical and histologic improvement on a strict gluten-free diet with relapse when gluten is reintroduced.

Etiology and Pathogenesis

- Celiac sprue affects 1 in 120 to 300 persons in both Europe and North America.
- Celiac sprue results from an inappropriate T-cell–mediated immune response against ingested gluten in genetically predisposed people.
- Individuals with celiac sprue express the HLA-DQ (α1*501, β1*02) heterodimer (HLA-DQ2), which preferentially presents gluten-derived gliadin peptides to stimulate intestinal mucosal T cells.
- The modification of gliadin by host tissue transglutaminase is detrimental in enhancing the gliadin-specific T-cell response.

- Diarrhea results from (a) changes in jejunal mucosal function; (b) secondary lactase deficiency, due to changes in jejunal brush border enzymatic function; (c) bile acid malabsorption stimulating fluid secretion in the colon, and (d) endogenous fluid secretion resulting from the crypt hyperplasia.

Clinical Manifestations

Onset may be in infancy or childhood with spontaneous remission during the second decade of life that may be either permanent or followed by recurrence years later. Alternatively, the symptoms may occur at any age throughout adulthood.

- In infants the introduction of cereals in the diet results in diarrhea, weight loss, abdominal distension, anemia, and poor growth.
- Children may present with recurrent abdominal pain, mild elevation in transaminases, recurrent aphthous stomatitis, arthralgia, defects in dental enamel, or behavioral disturbances such as depression.
- Adult-onset celiac disease may manifest as episodic or nocturnal diarrhea, flatulence, abdominal discomfort, bloating. Weight loss, and secondary lactose intolerance can occur. Malaise in the absence of anemia or recurrent aphthous stomatitis may be the sole symptom at presentation.
- Rare cases present with evidence of the depletion of a single nutrient (e.g., iron or folate deficiency, osteomalacia, edema from protein loss) and minimal GI symptoms.
- Dermatitis herpetiformis (DH) may be seen in a small percentage of patients with celiac disease. These pruritic, papulovesicular lesions are usually symmetrically located on the elbows, knees, sacrum, buttocks, face, and trunk and respond to dapsone.

Differential Diagnosis

Tropical sprue, eosinophilic enteritis, milk or soy protein intolerance in children, collagenous sprue, graft versus host disease, lymphoma, Whipple's disease, Crohn's disease, gastrinoma with acid hypersecretion. However, the presence of a characteristic histopathologic appearance that reverts toward normal following the initiation of a gluten-free diet establishes the diagnosis of celiac sprue.

Diagnosis

- Serology: The purpose of serology is to evaluate patients with suspected disease, monitor adherence and response to a gluten-free diet, screen patients with atypical, extraintestinal manifestations.
  - Immunoglobulin A (IgA) antiendomysial antibody: Moderately sensitive but highly specific for celiac disease
  - Antitissue transglutaminase IgA: Highly sensitive and highly specific

  - IgA antigliadin antibody: Moderately sensitive and moderately specific
  - Diagnosis in patients should be made with an IgA antiendomysial or Ig A anti tTG as these are highly specific and therefore have high positive predictive value.
  - Provided serologic assays on presentation have detected the presence of IgA antiendomysial or tTG antibodies, they should decline to undetectable 3 to 6 months after a gluten-free diet is started.
- EGD and biopsy
  - Biopsy is necessary to establish the diagnosis.
  - The changes seen on duodenal/jejunal biopsy and are restricted to the mucosa and consist of the following:
    Villous atrophy: Absence or reduced height of villi, resulting in a flat appearance; crypt hyperplasia; lymphocytic and plasma cell infiltration of the lamina propria

Failure to Respond to Gluten Restriction

- Inadvertent ingestion of gluten.
- Development of intestinal T-cell lymphoma. This diagnosis should be considered whenever a patient with celiac sprue previously doing well on a gluten-free diet is no longer responsive to gluten restriction.
- Collagenous sprue is a condition in which a layer of collagen-like material is present beneath the basement membrane.

Treatment

- Exclusion of all gluten from the diet.
- Patients with more severe involvement with celiac sprue may obtain temporary improvement with dietary lactose and fat restriction while awaiting the full effects of total gluten restriction.

Complications

An increased incidence of non-Hodgkin's lymphoma, metabolic bone disease, infertility, transaminitis and dermatitis herpetiformis. Celiac disease is associated with an increased incidence of type 1 diabetes mellitus and autoimmune thyroid disease as well as an association with IgA deficiency and Down syndrome.

Tropical Sprue

Tropical sprue is a diarrheal illness that occurs in endemic tropical areas manifesting as chronic diarrhea, steatorrhea, weight loss, and nutritional deficiency.

Epidemiology/Pathogenesis

- The etiology of tropical sprue is unknown but may be secondary to overgrowth of bacteria or their toxins as it does seem to improve with antibiotic therapy. The exact bacterial pathogens are unknown but *Klebsiella pneumoniae, Escherichia coli, Enterobacter cloacae* have been implicated.
- Tropical sprue is endemic to only certain tropical areas South India, the Philippines, Puerto Rico, and Haiti.

Clinical Manifestations

- Acute onset of steatorrhea
- Abdominal pain
- Weight loss
- B_{12}, folate deficiency, osteomalacia, edema from protein loss

Diagnosis

- Laboratory studies: Macrocytic anemia; elevated PT; PTT from vitamin K deficiency; low albumin; cholesterol and triglycerides; low B_{12} and folate. Stool should be examined for ova and parasites.
- EGD and biopsy: Histology is similar to celiac sprue with less villous atrophy and more mononuclear infiltrate but does not respond to gluten restriction.

Treatment

- Tetracycline with folate for 6 months.

Differential Diagnosis

Celiac sprue (B_{12} deficiency is not seen as the ileum is spared in celiac disease, histologically there is more villous atrophy in celiac disease), Whipple disease (B_{12} deficiency and ileal involvement are not seen, platelet antiserum (PAS)-positive macrophages and detection of *Tropheryma whipplei*)

Short Bowel Syndrome

Short bowel syndrome is defined as malabsorption that results from the resection of the small bowel.

Epidemiology/Pathogenesis

- Short bowel syndrome can occur at any age.
- Factors that determine both the type and degree of symptoms include the following:

- Segment of bowel resected, i.e., jejunum versus ileum. The ileum is the most adaptive part of the bowel, and therefore when the jejunum is resected the ileum takes over its function and absorbs nutrients and water. However, when the ileum is resected the colon is unable to absorb the fluid, nutrients (B_{12}) and bile salts resulting in steatorrhea.
- Length of the resected segment: Approximately 50% of the small bowel can be resected without significant compromise in fluid or water absorption.
- Integrity of the ileocecal valve: Removal of the valve results in an increased speed of transit and bacterial overgrowth.
- Concomitant removal of large intestine.
- Presence of residual disease in the remaining small or large intestine.

Clinical Manifestations

Diarrhea results from the following:

- Bile acids stimulate the colonic secretion of fluid and electrolytes.
- Bile salt malabsorption results in steatorrhea.
- Gastric acid inactivates pancreatic enzymes resulting in steatorrhea.
- Gastric hypersecretion also results in volume overload in a shortened small bowel.
- Absence of an ileocecal valve results in bacterial overgrowth.
- Lactose intolerance as a result of the removal of lactase-containing mucosa.
- Fat-soluble vitamin malabsorption (vitamin A, D, and E).
- Vitamin B_{12} malabsorption with ileal resection, consequent hyperhomocysteinemia can result in thrombosis.
- Dehydration and renal insufficiency.
- Gallstones secondary to super saturation of bile with cholesterol due to bile acid malabsorption.
- Nephrolithiasis with calcium oxalate stones due to an increase in oxalate absorption in the colon and hyperoxaluria.

Treatment

- Nutrition: In the initial stages with total parenteral nutrition and then oral feeding.
- Dietary modification: Lactose-free, low-fat and high-carbohydrate diet to minimize steatorrhea.
- Fat-soluble vitamins, folate, iron, vitamin B_{12}, calcium, and magnesium.
- Acid inhibition to inhibit gastric acid hypersecretion.
- Diarrhea: Antidiarrheals before meals.
- Cholestyramine and calcium may be used to treat hyperoxaluria in patients with renal stones.

- Intestinal transplantation for individuals with extensive intestinal resection who cannot be maintained without total parenteral nutrition (TPN).

Bacterial Overgrowth (Blind Loop Syndrome)

Bacterial overgrowth syndrome is a condition in which the presence of excessive bacteria in the small bowel results in malabsorption.

Etiology/Pathogenesis

Bacterial overgrowth occurs secondary to the following:

- Stasis caused by impaired peristalsis due to disorder in motility or anatomy
- Direct communication between the small and large intestine
- Immunodeficiency
- Increasing age

Clinical Manifestations

Manifestations of bacterial overgrowth syndromes are a direct consequence of the presence of increased amounts of a colonic-type bacterial flora in the small bowel.

- Bacterial deconjugation of bile acids results in the malabsorption of fat and fat-soluble vitamins (vitamin A, D, and E, vitamin K is produced by the bacteria). This manifests as steatorrhea, tetany, osteomalacia, night blindness.
- Bacterial enterotoxins produced in the colonized small bowel produce diarrhea without steatorrhea.
- Cobalamin deficiency due to consumption of dietary cobalamin by bacteria results in peripheral neuropathy, and macrocytic anemia with normal folate levels.
- Carbohydrate malabsorption secondary to the reduction of brush border disaccharidases. Lactase deficiency is the first to be affected, and abdominal pain, bloating, and diarrhea occur when consumed.

Diagnosis

- EGD: Jejunal aspirate with increased levels of colon type (aerobic and anaerobic) bacteria helps rule out other causes of malabsorption.
- Hydrogen breath test following lactulose administration resulting in an early peak in hydrogen followed by a late peak from colonic bacteria metabolism of lactulose.

Treatment

- Vitamin A and D supplementation.
- Surgical correction of strictures, diverticulum, or a proximal afferent loop.

- Promotility agents (e.g., metoclopramide, cisparide) used to treat motility disorders resulting in stasis.
- Broad-spectrum antibiotics: Amoxicillin/clavulonate, norfloxacin, metronidazole for 3 weeks or until symptoms remit. Recurrences are treated with antibiotics for 1 week per month whether or not symptoms are present.

Whipple Disease

Whipple's disease is a rare chronic multisystem disease caused by the bacteria *Tropheryma whipplei* associated with malabsorption, weight loss, arthralgia, central nervous system and cardiovascular manifestations. The disease predominantly affects middle-aged white males.

Clinical Manifestations

- Gastrointestinal: Diarrhea often with steatorrhea is the most common presenting complaint; abdominal bloating, cramps, distention, anorexia.
- Malabsorption results in vitamin deficiencies, hypoalbuminemia, and weight loss.
- Joint: Migratory large joint arthropathy.
- Central nervous system: Dementia, headache, muscle weakness, ophthalmoplegia, myoclonus, and insomnia. Convergent nystagmus associated with palatal, tongue, and mandibular movements called oculomasticatory myorhythmia is pathognomonic.
- Cardiovascular: Pericarditis or endocarditis affecting the mitral and aortic valves and fulminant myocarditis.
- Pulmonary: Chronic cough, pleuritic pain, pleural effusion, and mediastinal widening secondary to adenopathy.
- Ocular: Chronic uveitis with decreased acuity.
- Systemic: Fever, weight loss, anorexia.

Diagnosis

Whipple's disease should be suspected in patients with seronegative arthritis, with malabsorption and culture negative endocarditis. Biopsies from the small intestine demonstrate PAS-positive macrophages containing the characteristic small Gram-positive acid fast negative bacilli or by *T. whipplei* polymerase chain reaction (PCR).

Differential Diagnosis

PAS-positive macrophages containing *Mycobacterium avium* complex may be seen in patients with HIV/AIDS. However, unlike *M. avium*, which is acid fast, *T. whipplei* is not.

Treatment

Double-strength trimethoprim/sulfamethoxazole for 12 months.

TUMORS OF THE STOMACH AND SMALL BOWEL

Gastric Cancer

Gastric cancer is the second most common cause of cancer-related deaths in the world. Incidence is highest in Japan, China, South America, and Eastern Europe. There has been a rise in the incidence of adenocarcinoma of the proximal stomach and the gastroesophageal junction.

Etiology/Pathogenesis

Gastric cancers are predominantly adenocarcinomas (90%), the rest are non-Hodgkin's lymphomas or leiomyosarcomas. Adenocarcinomas are divided into intestinal and diffuse.

- Intestinal adenocarcinomas: Form ulcerative lesions in the distal stomach and on biopsy consist of cohesive cells forming gland-like tubular structures (Table 4-1).
- Diffuse adenocarcinomas: Cells lack cohesion and infiltrate the stomach wall without forming a discrete mass.

Molecular features of gastric cancer: Allelic deletions in tumor suppressor genes mutated in colon cancer (MCC), adenomatous polyposis coli (APC), and p53 have been identified. Intestinal-type

TABLE 4-1 Risk Factors for Gastric Cancer

Pre-existing Conditions:
1. Chronic atrophic gastritis
2. Pernicious anemia
3. *H. pylori*, Epstein–Barr virus infection
4. Barrett's esophagus
5. Menetrier disease
6. Gastric polyps
7. Obesity

Environmental Factors:
1. Low socioeconomic status
2. Cigarette smoking
3. Alcohol consumption
4. Diet: Salted, smoked, or preserved food, low fruit and vegetables

Genetic Factors:
1. Hereditary nonpolyposis colorectal cancer
2. *BRCA2* mutation
3. Family history of gastric cancer
4. Blood group A

adenocarcinomas have overexpression of protooncogenes for epidermal growth-factor receptor (erbB-2 and erbB-3). Diffuse-type adenocarcinomas have abnormalities of oncogenes for fibroblast growth-factor systems (K-sam).

Clinical Manifestations

- Asymptomatic in early stages.
- Gradual onset of upper abdominal discomfort aggravated by meals or constant pain.
- Dysphagia may be the main symptom associated with a lesion of the cardia.
- Vomiting may be seen if there is distal obstruction.
- Weight loss, anorexia, and nausea are frequently.
- Hematemesis or melena is reported by 20% of patients, but frank GI hemorrhage is rare.
- Penetration into the colon with resultant feculent emesis.
- Paraneoplastic conditions associated with gastric cancer are acanthosis nigricans, dermatomyositis, sudden development of seborrheic keratoses (sign of Leser–Trélat), membranous glomerulonephritis, microangiopathic hemolytic anemia, chronic intravascular coagulation leading to arterial and venous thrombi (Trousseau's syndrome).

Physical Examination

- Abdominal mass may occasionally be palpable.
- Left supraclavicular adenopathy (Virchow node).
- Periumbilical nodule (Sister Mary Joseph node).
- Frank peritoneal carcinomatosis and malignant ascites.
- Hepatomegaly with a hard palpable and nodular liver with metastases.
- Pelvic exam may reveal an enlarged ovary (Krukenberg's tumor), or a mass in the cul-de-sac (Blumer's shelf) (Table 4-2).

Diagnosis (Table 4-2)

- Upper gastrointestinal series: Diminished distensibility of the stomach, with diffuse infiltrative carcinoma. However, upper GI series is of limited sensitivity and specificity.
- EGD with biopsy: This is the test of choice as lesions can be visualized and biopsied.
- CT abdomen: To determine the extent of the primary tumor and presence of nodal or distant metastases, but may underestimate the depth of invasion.
- Endoscopic ultrasound: To determine the depth of tumor penetration and the presence of nodal metastases with accuracy higher than CT.

TABLE 4-2 Staging of Gastric Cancer

Primary Tumor (T)

TX: Primary tumor cannot be assessed
T0: No evidence of primary tumor
Tis: Carcinoma in situ: intraepithelial tumor without invasion of the lamina propria
T1: Tumor invades lamina propria or submucosa
T2: Tumor invades the muscularis propria or the subserosa*
T2a: Tumor invades muscularis propria
T2b: Tumor invades subserosa
T3: Tumor penetrates the serosa (visceral peritoneum) without invading adjacent structures**,***
T4: Tumor invades adjacent structures**,***

* [*Note: A tumor may penetrate the muscularis propria with extension into the gastrocolic or gastrohepatic ligaments, or into the greater or lesser omentum, without perforation of the visceral peritoneum covering these structures. In this case, the tumor is classified T2. If there is perforation of the visceral peritoneum covering the gastric ligaments or the omentum, the tumor should be classified T3.*]

** [*Note: The adjacent structures of the stomach include the spleen, transverse colon, liver, diaphragm, pancreas, abdominal wall, adrenal gland, kidney, small intestine, and retroperitoneum.*]

*** [*Note: Intramural extension to the duodenum or esophagus is classified by the depth of greatest invasion in any of these sites, including stomach.*]

Regional Lymph Nodes (N)

The regional lymph nodes are the perigastric nodes, found along the lesser and greater curvatures, and the nodes located along the left gastric, common hepatic, splenic, and celiac arteries. For pN, a regional lymphadenectomy specimen will ordinarily contain at least 15 lymph nodes. Involvement of other intra-abdominal lymph nodes, such as the hepatoduodenal, retropancreatic, mesentric, and para-aortic, is classified as distant metastasis.

NX: Regional lymph node(s) cannot be assessed
N0: No regional lymph node metastasis*
N1: Metastasis in one to six regional lymph nodes
N2: Metastasis in 7 to 15 regional lymph nodes
N3: Metastasis in more than 15 regional lymph nodes

* [*Note: A designation of pN0 should be used if all examined lymph nodes are negative, regardless of the total number removed and examined.*]

Distant Metastasis (M)

MX: Distant metastasis cannot be assessed
M0: No distant metastasis
M1: Distant metastasis

AJCC stage groupings

Stage 0
Tis, N0, M0
Stage IA
T1, N0, M0
Stage IB
T1, N1, M0
T2a, N0, M0
T2b, N0, M0

(*Continued*)

TABLE 4-2 Staging of Gastric Cancer (*Continued*)

Stage II
T1, N2, M0
T2a, N1, M0
T2b, N1, M0
T3, N0, M0
Stage IIIA
T2a, N2, M0
T2b, N2, M0
T3, N1, M0
T4, N0, M0
Stage IIIB
T3, N2, M0
Stage IV
T4, N1, M0
T4, N2, M0
T4, N3, M0
T1, N3, M0
T2, N3, M0
T3, N3, M0
Any T, any N, M1

With permission from *Stomach*. In: American Joint Committee on Cancer.: AJCC Cancer Staging Manual. 6th ed. New York, NY: Springer, 2002, p 101.

Treatment

- Surgery
  - Distal lesions in the antrum, pre-pyloric area are treated with subtotal gastrectomy and Billroth II or Roux-en-Y anastomosis (Fig. 4-3).
  - Midgastric and proximal lesions are treated with total gastrectomy and lymph node dissection. If the body or the tail of the pancreas is involved distal pancreatectomy can be performed together with a Roux-en-Y anastomosis (Fig. 4-4).
  - Distal esophageal involvement necessitates resection with the cardia and lesser curvature, and the remaining stomach is anastomosed to the mid-esophagus. If there is more extensive esophageal involvement, a near-complete esophagectomy is performed with colonic interposition.
  - Patients with incurable disease should be considered for palliative resection to provide relief from pain and obstruction provided they do not have ascites or extensive metastatic disease.
  - Laser ablation of tumor tissue can be effective, although relief is transient, and repeated treatments are required.
  - Adjuvant chemoradiotherapy is controversial.

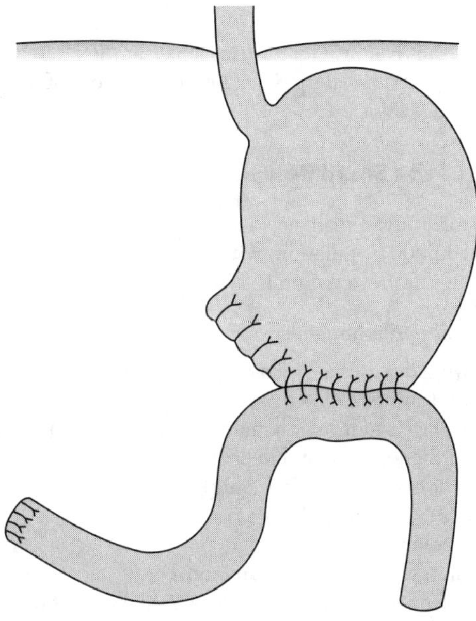

Figure 4-3 • Billroth II reconstruction after antral gastric cancer resection. (From Karp S, Morris J, Soybel, D. *Blueprints surgery.* 3rd ed. Oxford: Blackwell; 2004, with permission).

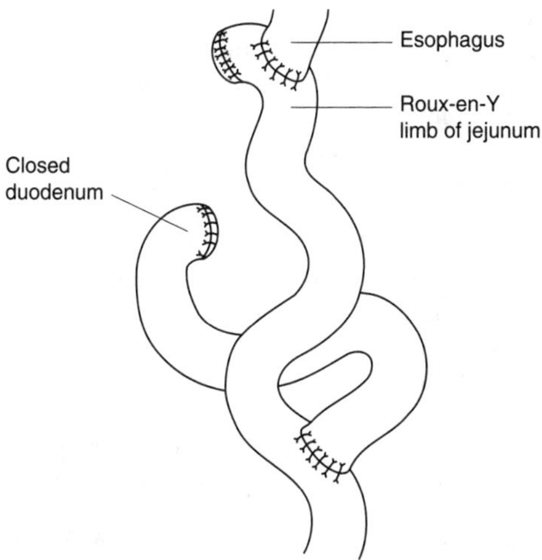

Figure 4-4 • Roux-en-Y esophagojejunostomy reconstruction after total gastrectomy. (From Karp S, Morris J, Soybel, D. *Blueprints surgery.* 3rd ed. Oxford: Blackwell; 2004, with permission.)

Prognosis

The overall survival rate for gastric cancer in the United States is 10%. The 5-year survival for Stage I is 70%, Stage II 30%, Stage III 10%, and Stage IV is 0%.

Tumors of the Small Bowel

Primary small bowel malignancies are rare with an incidence is 1 to 2 per 100,000 population, with a slight male predominance; the mean age at presentation is 57 years.

Epidemiology/Pathogenesis

The following diseases are all associated with an increased risk of small bowel tumors:

- Peutz–Jeghers syndrome (hamartomatous polyps occurring primarily in the jejunum and ileum)
- Crohn's disease (adenocarcinoma)
- Gardner's syndrome (adenoma)
- Familial colonic polyposis (adenoma)
- Celiac disease (lymphoma, carcinoma)
- Immunodeficiency states and autoimmune disorders (lymphoma)

Malignant Small Bowel Tumors

There are four main histologic types of malignant small bowel tumors: adenocarcinoma, carcinoid, lymphoma, and sarcoma.

- Adenocarcinoma
  - Frequently associated with familial adenomatous polyposis (FAP). Tumors are predominantly located in the duodenum and are mainly periampullary, but adenocarcinomas arising from Crohn's disease are predominantly ileal.
  - Usually presents between the ages of 50 and 70 years, with a male predominance.
  - May present as occult GI bleeding or chronic anemia.
  - Abdominal pain and intestinal obstruction can be caused by progression of an apple core or by a large intraluminal polypoid mass.
  - Anorexia and weight loss are frequently seen.
- Carcinoid tumors
  - Carcinoids are indolent neuroendocrine tumors arising from the Kulchitsky cell, an enterochromaffin cell located in the crypts of Lieberkuhn.
  - Carcinoids are most commonly located in the appendix, followed by the small bowel and rectum.
  - Clinically significant carcinoids are most commonly located in the ileum.

- The age at presentation ranges from 20 to 80 years with the highest incidence in the fifth to sixth decade.
- Tumors are usually intramucosal; however, infiltration of the serosa results in an intense desmoplastic reaction with shortening and thickening of the mesentery and resultant abdominal pain.
- Carcinoids tumors secrete serotonin, but can also secrete corticotropin, dopamine, substance P, histamine, neurotensin, prostaglandins, and kallikrein. Carcinoid syndrome is seen when these products are able to gain access to systemic circulation and avoid metabolism in the liver such as with liver metastases, an extraintestinal primary carcinoid (such as in the lung or testes), or retroperitoneal disease.
- Carcinoids are classified according to their presumed derivation from different embryonic divisions of the gut and their histologic characteristics. Foregut carcinoids most commonly originate in the lungs, bronchi, or stomach. Midgut carcinoids in the small intestine, appendix, and proximal large bowel; and hindgut carcinoids in the distal colon and rectum.
- The distinction between benign and malignant carcinoids is based on the presence or absence of metastasis rather than on histology alone.
- The 5-year survival rates are 55% overall, 65% for local disease, 64% for regional disease, and 36% for metastatic disease (Modlin IM et al.)

• Lymphoma
  - Small bowel lymphomas are categorized into primary small bowel lymphoma (PSBL) and immuno proliferative small intestinal disease (IPSID).
  - PSBL occurs predominantly in adult males in the seventh decade; IPSID occurs in the second to third decade.
  - Predisposing conditions for PSBL (which are predominantly T cell) are autoimmune diseases, immunodeficiency states, postradiation therapy, Crohn's disease, and celiac sprue.
  - IPSID occurs in areas of poor hygiene in the Middle East, Southeast Asia, South America, are predominantly B cell, and can be eradicated with antibiotics.
  - B-cell lymphomas most often involving the GI tract consist of the MALT type (mucosa-associated lymphoid tissue), mantle cell, Burkitt's, and Burkitt-like variants. MALT type tumors (also called extranodal marginal zone B-cell lymphoma of MALT type in the REAL/WHO classification) occur most often in the stomach. Mantle cell lymphoma has a predilection for the colon and small intestine.
  - The 5-year survival ranges from 20% to 30%.

- Sarcoma
  - Sarcomas represent approximately 10% of small bowel neoplasms, and are most commonly located in the jejunum, ileum, and in Meckel's diverticulum.
  - The most common type is a leiomyosarcoma (75%) followed by fibrosarcoma, liposarcoma, and angiosarcoma.
  - Small intestinal sarcomas are large tumors and can exceed 5 cm in diameter. They are typically slow growing and enlarge extraluminaly.
  - Patients present with abdominal pain, weight loss, bleeding, or perforation. Palpable mass and obstruction are late symptoms.
  - Sarcomas can metastasize hematogenously and present with disease in the liver, lungs, or bones.
- Metastases: The small bowel is the most common site of gastrointestinal metastatic melanoma. Other primary tumors can involve the small bowel by hematogenous spread (e.g., kidney, lung, and breast cancer) or directly (e.g., cervical, ovarian, and colon cancer).

Benign Lesions of the Small Bowel

Include adenomas, lipomas, leiomyomas, and hemangiomas. Villous adenomas carry a significant potential for malignant transformation. FAP, a hereditary cancer syndrome, or its attenuated forms can present with duodenal polyps, and colonoscopy should be performed to rule out colonic polyps and cancer.

Clinical Manifestations

Clinical presentations of benign and malignant lesions are similar.

- Asymptomatic: Many patients with malignant tumors are asymptomatic until the tumor has spread beyond the stage of surgical cure.
- Intermittent abdominal pain is the most common presenting symptom with anorexia and weight loss, intussusception, occult bleeding, palpable abdominal mass or obstruction.
- Perforation and hematochezia are rare.
- Carcinoid syndrome may present with abdominal cramping, watery diarrhea, flushing, sweating, hypotension, wheezing, dyspnea from right heart failure due to tricuspid regurgitation or pulmonic stenosis caused by endocardial fibrosis or, more rarely, from bronchospasm. Flushing is precipitated by exercise, alcohol, blue cheese, chocolate.
- Carcinoid crisis is usually precipitated by a specific event such as anesthesia, surgery, or chemotherapy. The manifestations include an intense flush, diarrhea, tachycardia, hypertension or hypotension, bronchospasm, and alteration of mental status. The symptoms are usually refractory to fluid resuscitation and administration of vasopressors.

Diagnosis

- Small bowel series: Upper GI series with small bowel follow through (UGI/SBFT) has low sensitivity.
- Computed tomography: CT can detect local and regional spread for staging.
- Enteroclysis: Enteroclysis is a double-contrast study performed by passing a tube into the proximal small bowel and injecting barium and methylcellulose. This technique has a higher sensitivity to UGI/SBFT.
- CT enteroclysis combines the advantages of CT and enteroclysis; its accuracy for diagnosing small bowel neoplasms is still being determined.
- Capsule endoscope may also be used to visualize the small bowel but does not allow for biopsies.
- Upper GI endoscopy or enteroscopy (with a pediatric colonoscope or enteroscope) may allow visualization of the proximal 60 cm of jejunum and allows for biopsies to be taken.
- Exploratory laparotomy is used to establish the diagnosis of a small bowel tumor if there is high index of suspicion and negative workup.
- 24-h urinary excretion of hydroxyindole acetic acid (HIAA): In patients with suspected carcinoids. 5-HIAA is the end product of serotonin metabolism and is highly specific but can be misleading if certain foods and drugs are not avoided.
- Radionuclide scans using radiolabeled (iodine-131 or -121) metaiodobenzylguanidine (MIBG), which is taken up by the tumor and stored, can be used to identify primary or metastatic carcinoid tumors.
- Radionuclide imaging using indium-111 octreotide is useful for localization of carcinoids before surgery and to predict response to octreotide therapy.

Treatment

- Malignant tumors: Pancreaticoduodenectomy may be required for tumors in the second or third portion of the duodenum; a right colectomy is indicated for tumors of the distal ileum.
  - Adjuvant chemotherapy similar to that used to treat colorectal cancer (based on fluorouracil, 5-FU) has been used for adenocarcinomas.
  - Small bowel metastases are treated with limited resection for palliation. Aggressive resection is indicated in patients with malignant melanomas.
- Benign tumors: Tubular adenomas have a low malignant potential and can be treated with polypectomy or simple local resection.
  - Villous adenomas have a malignant potential similar to colonic adenomas. Endoscopic polypectomy or simple resection is sufficient if no invasive carcinoma is found in the specimen.

Periampullary adenomas containing areas of malignant growth still require radical surgery.
- Leiomyomas are difficult to differentiate from leiomyosacrcomas. Mitotic index (MI), defined as the number of mitoses per 50 high power fields, is used to guide management. Leiomyomas with MI ≥ 2 should be considered for close follow-up and further therapy.
- Lipomas have no malignant potential and are excised if symptomatic.
- Peutz–Jeghers syndrome is an inherited disorder characterized by mucocutaneous melanotic pigmentation and gastrointestinal hamartomatous polyps with no malignant potential. Treatment is limited to the segment responsible for symptoms.

Acute Small Bowel Obstruction

Epidemiology/Pathogenesis

- The most frequent causes of small bowel obstruction are postoperative adhesions and hernias, which cause extrinsic compression of the intestine.
- The small bowel proximal to the obstruction begins to dilate because of the failure of passage of intestinal secretions and swallowed air, fermentation by bacteria, and decreased absorptive capacity due to edema.
- Strangulation occurs when gut edema and increased intraluminal pressure compromise perfusion resulting in necrosis and perforation (Table 4-3).

Clinical Manifestations (Fig. 4-5)

- Periumbilical, crampy abdominal pain, which later becomes constant.
- Nausea and vomiting are more severe in proximal obstruction, as compared to distal obstruction. The vomitus becomes more

TABLE 4-3 Causes of Small Bowel Obstruction
Benign strictures: Postoperative adhesions, Crohn's disease, ischemia, radiation
Neoplasm: Intraluminal or extrinsic compression
Hernias: Femoral, inguinal, ventral
Intussusception
Meckel diverticulum
Volvulus
Gallstone ileus
Bezoar
Superior mesenteric artery syndrome

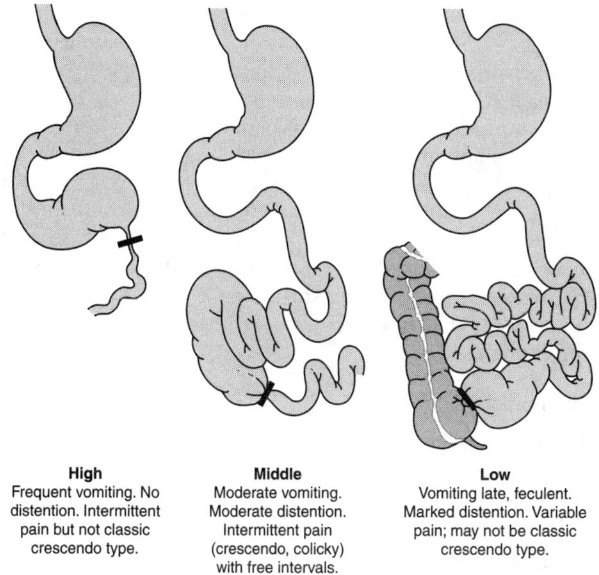

High
Frequent vomiting. No distention. Intermittent pain but not classic crescendo type.
Middle
Moderate vomiting. Moderate distention. Intermittent pain (crescendo, colicky) with free intervals.
Low
Vomiting late, feculent. Marked distention. Variable pain; may not be classic crescendo type.

Figure 4-5 • Variable manifestations of small bowel obstruction depending on the level of blockage. (From Karp S, Morris J, Soybel, D. *Blueprints surgery.* 3rd ed. Oxford: Blackwell; 2004, with permission.)

feculent as obstruction continues secondary to bacterial overgrowth.

- Abdominal distention is more pronounced in distal small bowel obstruction as the proximal intestine dilates.
- Patients may pass gas and stool 12 to 24 h after the onset, as the colon distal to obstruction empties following which patients develop obstipation.
- Dehydration, electrolyte abnormalities, and renal failure can result.

Physical Examination

- Inspection: Abdominal distension, surgical scars, femoral and inguinal hernia.
- Auscultation: High-pitched or hypoactive bowel sounds
- Palpation: Guarding, rigidity, and rebound suggest the development of peritonitis; an abdominal mass may be palpable.
- Percussion: Tympanitic secondary to air-filled loops of bowel.

Diagnosis

- History of previous intra-abdominal surgeries, previous episodes of small bowel obstruction, inflammatory bowel disease, and cancer screening.

- Laboratory data: Electrolyte abnormalities secondary to dehydration may be seen as well as an elevated BUN/ creatinine due to prerenal renal failure. Metabolic alkalosis from repeated emesis or an anion gap metabolic acidosis from lactate due to ischemic bowel. An elevated white blood count may also be seen.
- Radiology, upright kidney, ureter, bladder (KUB): Multiple air fluid levels and distended loops of small bowel suggest a small bowel obstruction or paralytic ileus. If gas is present in the rectum, it suggests that the obstruction is partial. Biliary gas and an opacity in the right lower quadrant suggest gallstone ileus.
- CT abdomen: Can confirm the presence of a partial or complete obstruction and determine the point of obstruction and the etiology.

Differential Diagnosis

Paralytic ileus and intestinal pseudo-obstruction.

Treatment

- Nil per oral (NPO).
- Nasogastric decompression.
- Monitor volume status and urine output.
- Assess degree of dehydration; correct and replace electrolyte derangements.
- Intravenous fluids.
- Urgent surgical management is necessary for patients with a complete small bowel obstruction, a closed loop obstruction strangulation, ischemia or perforation and should be considered in patients with a partial small bowel obstruction which fails to resolve.

Chapter 5

Diseases of the Colon and Rectum

Irritable Bowel Syndrome

Irritable bowel syndrome (IBS) is characterized by chronic abdominal pain and altered bowel habits (constipation or diarrhea) that occur without an underlying organic pathology. IBS is the most frequently diagnosed gastrointestinal (GI) disorder.

Epidemiology/Pathogenesis

- Altered bowel motility, visceral hypersensitivity, psychosocial factors, imbalance in neurotransmitters, and infection have all been proposed as possible mechanisms.
- IBS predominantly affects younger patients with a 2:1 female predominance.

Clinical Manifestations

- Abdominal pain: Predominantly left lower quadrant cramping. Pain is exacerbated with emotional stress and food and relieved with defecation.
- Altered bowel habits: Diarrhea, constipation, or alternating diarrhea and constipation with interspersed periods of normal bowel habits.
- Diarrhea: Frequent small to moderate-volume loose stools often associated with mucus. Diarrhea is aggravated by meals but characteristically patients have no nocturnal symptoms. Despite the passage of stool, patients with diarrhea have a sense of incomplete evacuation.
- Constipation: Stools are often hard and pellet shaped with a sense of incomplete evacuation even when the rectum is empty.
- Abdominal bloating, flatulence, and belching are frequently seen (Table 5-1).

Differential Diagnosis

Malabsorption, lactose intolerance, ulcerative colitis, Crohn's disease, diverticulitis, infectious colitis, and bowel obstruction.

Diagnosis

- Laboratory tests: Complete blood count, complete metabolic panel, thyroid-stimulating hormone (TSH), and antitissue transglutaminase antibody (anti-TTG)

TABLE 5-1 ROME III Diagnostic Criteria* for Irritable Bowel Syndrome

Recurrent abdominal pain or discomfort ** at least 3 days per month in the last 3 months associated with *2 or more* of the following:

1. Improvement with defecation
2. Onset associated with a change in frequency of stool
3. Onset associated with a change in form (appearance) of stool

** Criteria fulfilled for the last 3 months with symptom onset at least 6 months prior to diagnosis.** Discomfort means an uncomfortable sensation not described as pain. In pathophysiology research and clinical trials, a pain/discomfort frequency of at least 2 days a week during screening evaluation for subject eligibility.*

Reproduced with permission from Longstreth G, Thompson WG, Chey W, et al. Functional Bowel Disorders. In: *Gastroenterology* 2006;130(5):1480–1491. Copyright 2006 by the American Gastroenterological Association Institute.

- Endoscopy: Flexible sigmoidoscopy with biopsy in patients <50 years old with no alarm symptoms, but colonoscopy with biopsy and CT abdomen is necessary in patients with alarm symptoms.

Treatment

- Dietary modification: An empiric trial of a lactose-free diet.
- Diarrhea-predominant IBS:
  - Antidiarrheal agents such as loperamide and diphenoxylate.
  - Cholestyramine binds bile acids that may be responsible for increased secretion and decreased absorption of water in the colon.
  - Antibiotics have been used in refractory cases and may decrease diarrhea by altering the intestinal flora.
- Constipation-predominant IBS:
  - Increased dietary fiber.
  - Laxatives including osmotic laxatives (lactulose and sorbitol), magnesium-containing laxatives, or polyethylene glycol solution can be used to treat constipation.
  - 5 HT4 agonists such as tegaserod increase colonic motility and are used in patients with constipation-predominant IBS. Tegaserod can be used only in women.
- Abdominal pain:
  - Antispasmodic agents (anticholinergic agents, e.g., dicyclomine; smooth muscle relaxants, e.g., mebeverine).
  - Nitrates.
  - Tricyclic antidepressants may be of benefit in the treatment of patients with IBS and neuropathic pain. They have not been shown to be effective in the improvement of IBS symptoms.

  - Refractory pain: Nonsteroidal anti-inflammatories (NSAIDs) and opioid analogues.
- Behavior modification and biofeedback may be of particular utility in patients whose symptoms are aggravated by stress.

INFLAMMATORY BOWEL DISEASE

Crohn's Disease

Crohn's disease is characterized by transmural mucosal inflammation of any part of the GI tract from the mouth to the anus.

Etiology/Pathogenesis

Possible etiologies include:

- Inappropriate and prolonged immune response to normal dietary or luminal flora.
- Genetic factors:
  - Family history of inflammatory bowel disease (IBD) is the most important risk factor.
  - Frameshift mutation in the *NOD2* gene is associated with 20-fold or greater increase in susceptibility. However, it is estimated that only 15% of patients with Crohn's disease have mutations in *NOD2*.
- Environmental factors:
  - NSAIDs by altering the intestinal barrier can precipitate flares.
  - High level of sanitation in childhood is associated with an increased incidence of Crohn's disease, presumably from an exaggerated immune response to antigens that an individual may have been normally exposed to earlier in life.
  - Smoking may be protective against ulcerative colitis but increases the risk of Crohn's disease.

Clinical Manifestations

Crohn's disease can involve the entire GI tract from mouth to perianal area (Fig. 5-1). There are three patterns of involvement: ileocolitis (45%), ileal (30%), and colon (25%).

- Crampy abdominal pain is a common manifestation.
- Weight loss secondary to malabsorption or decreased intake.
- Diarrhea occurs secondary to inflammation of the bowel with decreased reabsorption of fluid; bile salt malabsorption secondary to inflammation of the terminal ileum or after resection results in fat malabsorption; bacterial overgrowth from small bowel strictures or enterocolic fistula with colonization of colonic bacteria also results in malabsorption and enteroenteric fistulae result in loss of absorptive epithelium.

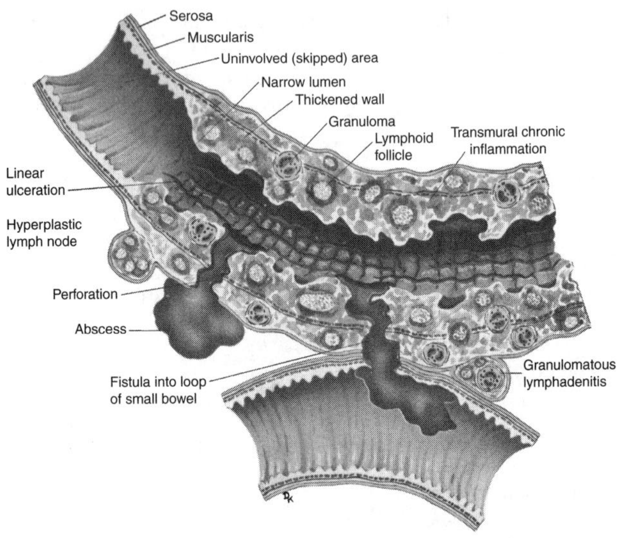

Figure 5-1 • Crohn's disease. A schematic representation of the major features of Crohn's disease in the small intestine.

- Low-grade fever.
- Hemoccult-positive stools may be seen but gross bleeding is rare.
- Fibrotic strictures of the small bowel and less frequently the colon may result in obstruction.
- Perianal skin tags, anal fissures, fistulae, and perirectal abscesses. Extraintestinal manifestations include the following:
  - Joints: Peripheral arthritis, which primarily involves large joints knee, hip, ankle, elbow, spares the hands. Peripheral arthritis parallels gut involvement. Ankylosing spondylitis does not parallel bowel disease. Patients present with lower back pain and morning stiffness. Osteoporosis secondary to malabsorption, inflammation, medications (steroids, cyclosporine).
  - Skin: Erythema nodosum and pyoderma gangrenosum.
  - Renal: Calcium oxalate stones from increased gut reabsorption of oxalate.
  - Eye: Uveitis and episcleritis.
  - Liver: Fatty liver, chronic active hepatitis, sclerosing cholangitis, and gallstones.
  - Venous and arterial thromboembolism with an increase in procoagulants and decrease in antithrombin III.
- Sinus tracts leading to fistula formation, bowel wall perforation, or peritonitis.

- Enteroenteric fistulae.
- Enterocutaneous fistula.
- Enterovesical fistulae resulting in recurrent urinary tract infections and air in the urine (pneumaturia).
- Retroperitoneal fistula may lead to a psoas abscesses and/or ureteral obstruction with–hydronephrosis.
- Enterovaginal fistula may present with passage of gas or feces through the vagina.

Diagnosis

- Family history of IBD makes the diagnosis more likely.
- Physical examination may be nonspecific or patients may have features of Crohn's disease with perianal skin tags, sinus tracts, and a palpable abdominal mass.
- Colonoscopy with biopsy
  - Focal ulcerations adjacent to areas of normal appearing mucosa along with polypoid mucosal changes that give a classic cobblestone appearance.
  - Skip areas consisting of segments of normal-appearing bowel interrupted by large areas of obvious disease; in contrast to continuous small bowel involvement in patients with ulcerative colitis.
  - Pseudopolyps secondary to inflammation.
  - Biopsy reveals focal ulcerations with acute and chronic inflammation.
  - Granulomas may be present in one third of cases and are diagnostic of the Crohn's disease once an infectious etiology can be excluded.
- Upper GI series with small bowel follow through
  - Narrowing of the lumen with nodularity and ulceration.
  - "String" sign refers to the narrowing of the bowel lumen in patients with advanced disease or spasm.
  - Narrowing of the gastric antrum and stricturing with gastroduodenal involvement.
- Antibody tests
  - Used to differentiate patients with ulcerative colitis and Crohn's disease in whom the diagnosis in uncertain; should only be used as an adjunct to endoscopy and biopsy. Ruemmele et al. demonstrated that patients with Crohn's disease are more likely to test positive for anti-*Saccharomyces cerevisiae* antibodies (ASCA) and negative to pANCA (perinuclear antineutrophil cytoplasmic antibody) and that patients who test positive for atypical pANCA (i.e., not directed against myeloperoxidase) and negative for ASCA were more likely to have ulcerative colitis.

- Capsule endoscopy is contraindicated in patients with strictures because the capsule may not be able to pass the stricture, necessitating surgery for retrieval.
- In up to 15% of patients with IBD involving only the colon, Crohn's disease cannot be distinguished from ulcerative colitis, and a diagnosis of indeterminate colitis is made.

Complications

Stricture, obstruction, hemorrhage, fistula, perforation, abscess, toxic megacolon, and increased risk of colorectal cancer. Surveillance for colorectal cancer in Crohn's colitis is the same as that for ulcerative colitis outlined in the next section.

Ulcerative Colitis

Ulcerative colitis is characterized by recurring episodes of mucosal inflammation that is confined to the colon. It starts in the rectum and extends proximally to involve other portions of the colon.

Clinical Manifestations

The initial episode of ulcerative colitis is limited to the rectum or distal colon in one third of patients, to the left colon up to the splenic flexure in one third, and most of the remaining patients have pancolitis.

- Mild disease: Colitis is confined to the rectum or rectosigmoid. Patients have gradual onset of bloody diarrhea with less than four small loose stools per day and mild anemia, but are afebrile.
- Moderate disease: Colitis involves the distal colon extending proximally to involve the left colon and up to 10 episodes of diarrhea per day associated with mild anemia, low-grade fever, and moderate abdominal pain.
- Severe or fulminant ulcerative colitis: Patients present with pancolitis and have more than 10 episodes of diarrhea in 24 h associated with severe abdominal pain, high fever, and anemia.
- Extraintestinal manifestations are common to both ulcerative colitis and Crohn's colitis and have been outlined previously (Fig. 5-2).

Diagnosis

The diagnosis of ulcerative colitis is established by the characteristic history with the following studies:

- CT abdomen and pelvis: May show marked thickening of the bowel wall and is of value in determining the extent of colitis.
- Flexible sigmoidoscopy and biopsy: Endoscopy shows erythematous friable mucosa, petechiae, exudates with continuous

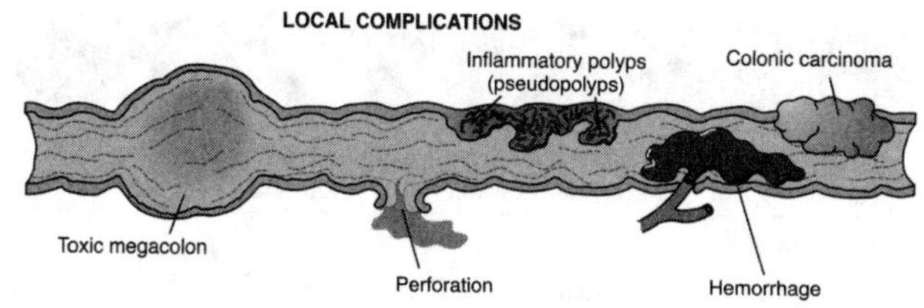

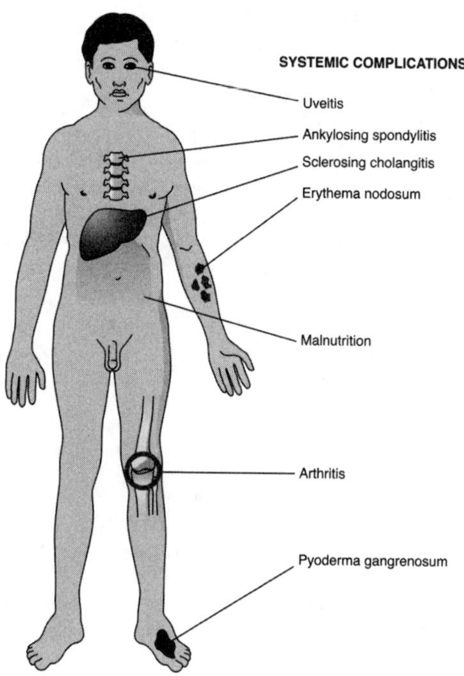

Figure 5-2 • Complications of ulcerative colitis.

ulcerations, and pseudopolyps. Biopsy reveals crypt abscesses and chronic changes including branching of crypts, atrophy of glands, and loss of mucin in goblet cells.

Differential Diagnosis

Crohn's colitis, infectious colitis: *Yesinia* (ileal), *Salmonella, Shigella, Campylobacter* (colitis), small bowel lymphoma, ileocecal tuberculosis, Bechet syndrome, amebiasis, collagenous colitis, and ischemic colitis (Table 5-2).

TABLE 5-2 Distinctive Features of Crohn's Disease and Ulcerative Colitis*

Features	Crohn's Disease (Small Intestine)	Crohn's Disease (Large Intestine)	Ulcerative Colitis
MACROSCOPIC			
Bowel region	Ileum +/– colon**	Colon +/– ileum	Colon only
Distribution	Skip lesions	Skip lesions	Diffuse
Stricture	Early	Variable	Late
Wall appearance	Thickened	Variable	Thin
Dilation	No	Yes	Yes
MICROSCOPIC			
Pseudopolyps	None to slight	Marked	Marked
Ulcers	Deep linear	Deep linear	Superficial
Lymphoid Reaction	Marked	Marked	Mild
Fibrosis	Marked	Moderate	Mild
Serositis	Marked	Variable	Mild to None
Granulomas	Yes (40–60%)	Yes (40–60%)	No
Fistulae/Sinuses	Yes	Yes	No
CLINICAL			
Fat/vitamin malabsorption	Yes	Yes if ileum	No
Malignant potential	Yes	Yes	Yes
Response to surgery+	Poor	Fair	Good

** Not all features present in a single case*

*** Crohn's disease can occur elsewhere in the small intestine as well*

+ Based on the likelihood of disease recurrence following surgical removal of a diseased segment

Reprinted with permission from Kumar, Cotran and Robbins, *Basic Pathology*, Chapter 15 The Oral Cavity and gastrointestinal tract, Sixth Edition, W.B. Saunders.

Complications

- Strictures occur late in the course of ulcerative colitis, and patients present with diarrhea and fecal incontinence.
- Fulminant colitis occurs in 10% of patients with ulcerative colitis; up to one fourth of these patients develop toxic megacolon.
- Toxic megacolon.
- Colorectal cancer in patients with longstanding disease.

Toxic Megacolon

- Toxic megacolon is the dilatation of the colon when inflammation extends beyond the submucosa into the muscularis mucosa.
- Toxic megacolon may result as a complication of ulcerative colitis or infectious colitis secondary to *Salmonella*, *Shigella*, *Campylobacter*, *Clostridium difficile*, or cytomegalovirus colitis.

Clinical Manifestations

- Fever, tachycardia (heart rate >120 bpm), leukocytosis (WBC >10,500 cell/mm^3), anemia, and signs of systemic toxicity; hypotension, dehydration, electrolyte abnormalities, mental status changes may be present.
- Physical examination is notable for abdominal distension with hypoactive bowel sounds and tenderness to palpation over the colon.
- Criteria for diagnosis include radiographic distension in addition to three of four clinical features and one sign of systemic toxicity (hypotension, dehydration, electrolyte abnormalities, or mental status changes).

Treatment

- Nil per oral (NPO).
- Nasogastric decompression.
- Intravenous fluids to replete volume and electrolyte loss.
- Roll patients supine to prone every 2 h to help redistribute the gas.
- Broad-spectrum antibiotics.
- Serial radiographs of the abdomen to monitor the course.
- Parenteral steroids.
- Patients who fail to respond to therapy in 48 h should be considered for proctocolectomy.
- Perforation occurs in patients with toxic megacolon and is more likely to occur with the first attack of ulcerative colitis due to the absence of associated wall fibrosis.

Colorectal Cancer

- Colorectal cancer (CRC) risk depends on the duration and extent of the disease.
- Incidence increases 8 to 10 years after the onset of disease in those patients with disease beyond the splenic flexure with an increase of 0.5% per year between 10 and 20 years and 1% per year thereafter. Risk of CRC is greatest in patients with pancolitis.
- Recommended surveillance is with colonoscopy and biopsy (4 quadrant every 10 cm) every 1 to 2 years after 8 years in patients with pancolitis and after 15 years in patients with left-sided colitis.

Treatment of Ulcerative Colitis and Crohn's Disease

5-ASA (5-aminosalicylic acid) Compounds

- 5-Aminosalicylate acts by scavenging free radicals inhibiting neutrophil respiratory burst and inhibiting 5-lipooxygenase, thereby blocking the synthesis of prostaglandins and leukotrienes.

- Sulfasalzine inhibits the activation of nuclear factor-κB that is critical to the expression of genes involved in the inflammatory response.
- Side effects: Nausea, vomiting, anorexia, headache, sperm abnormalities, hemolysis, and hepatitis.

Antibiotics

- Metronidazole has been used in the treatment of patients with perianal fistulas and with colonic Crohn's colitis. Ciprofloxacin has been shown to be equivalent.
- Antibiotics have no proven benefit in acute ulcerative colitis; however, patients with fulminant ulcerative colitis with fever/leukocytosis and peritoneal signs need to be covered with broad-spectrum antibiotics.
- Side effects: Metallic taste, peripheral neuropathy with numbness and burning of the feet; ingestion of alcohol with metronidazole results in a disulfuram-like reaction.
- Administration of beneficial bacterial species (probiotics), poorly absorbed dietary oligosaccharides (prebiotics), or combined probiotics and prebiotics (synbiotics) can restore a predominance of beneficial *Lactobacillus* and *Bifidobacterium* species. Probiotics have been used to treat active Crohn's disease and pouchitis.

Corticosteroids

- Steroids are indicated in the induction of remission in ulcerative colitis flares but have no proven benefit in maintenance.
- Hydrocortisone suppositories are indicated in patients with proctitis; retention enemas are indicated for patients with distal ulcerative colitis.
- Oral prednisone or prednisolone is used for induction of remission in moderately severe ulcerative colitis or Crohn's disease.
- Oral budesonide can be used in patients with distal ileal and right-sided colonic disease. As a result of its high first-pass metabolism, it has fewer side effects than prednisone.
- Intravenous steroids are indicated in hospitalized patients.
- Side effects: Acne, centripetal obesity, striae, moon facies, buffalo hump, cataracts, increased risk of infections, hyperglycemia, growth failure, avascular necrosis of the femur, osteoporosis, and adrenal insufficiency.
- All patients started on steroids should be placed on calcium and vitamin D, and based on the duration of steroids prophylaxis for *Pneumocystis carinii* pneumonia (*Pneumocystis jiroveci* pneumonia) should be considered.

Immunosuppressants

- These agents are generally appropriate for patients with ulcerative colitis or Crohn's disease who are steroid refractory or steroid dependent.
- Azathioprine or its active metabolite 6-mercaptopurine (6-MP).
  - Patients have a delayed response and improvement in symptoms is seen 2 to 5 months after initiation of azathioprine. Steroid therapy is therefore necessary during this time and gradual reduction of azathioprine dose can be started 2 to 3 months after starting azathioprine.
  - Side effects: Leukopenia, pancreatitis, allergy, hepatotoxicity and infections. Toxicity is dose-dependent thiopurine methyltransferase activity that converts 6-MP into its inactive metabolite 6-thioguanine (6-TG). As there is significant genetic polymorphism for thiopurine methyltransferase (TMPT) genotyping or measurement of 6-TG levels can be used to optimize dosing.
- Methotrexate
  - Used in patients with Crohn's disease who do not tolerate or are unresponsive to azathioprine or 6-MP or in patients with Crohn's related arthropathy. There are no data to support the use of methotrexate in ulcerative colitis.
  - Side effects: Bone marrow suppression, interstitial pneumonitis, and hepatic fibrosis. Bone marrow suppression with methotrexate can be minimized with folate. Toxicity is increased with renal failure and concomitant use of trimethoprim/sulfamethoxazole.
- Cyclosporine
  - Cyclosporine is used in patients with steroid-refractory severe ulcerative colitis in whom colectomy is being considered.
  - The advantage of cyclosporine is that its onset of action is within days.
  - Intravenous cyclosporine is started with 6-MP and then switched to oral cyclosporine for 3 months and then discontinued.
  - Side effects: Renal insufficiency, seizures in patients with low cholesterol levels, hypertension, bone marrow suppression, hepatotoxicity, hair growth. Patients should be started on prophylaxis against *Pneumocystis carinii* pneumonia (*Pneumocystis jiroveci* pneumonia).

Infliximab

- Infliximab is a chimeric mouse/human monoclonal antibody against tumor necrosis factor alpha (TNF-α) used in moderate to severe Crohn's disease that is steroid refractory.
- Infliximab also has a role in healing fistulae in Crohn's disease.

- Problems associated with infliximab are a shortening in the duration of response with repeated doses and increased toxicity with repeat doses.
- Patients starting infliximab must have a Mantoux test with purified protein derivative and, if positive, treated with isoniazid (INH) prior to starting therapy.
- Side effects: Infections, lymphoma, tuberculosis, and allergic reactions.

Surgery

- Indications in ulcerative colitis
  - Intractable disease with failure to respond after 7 to 10 days of cyclosporine therapy
  - Perforation
  - Toxic megacolon
  - Hemorrhage
  - Systemic complications
  - Dysplasia/cancer
- Indications in Crohn's disease
  - Failure to respond to medical management
  - Perforation
  - Stricture
  - Fistulae
  - Dysplasia/cancer

Colonic Obstruction

Colonic obstruction is predominantly caused by colon cancer; additional causes include extrinsic tumor compression (lymph nodes, metastatic disease), volvulus, and adhesions.

Volvulus

Volvulus is the twisting of a part of the bowel on itself around a fixed point of attachment. The most common sites in the colon are the sigmoid colon and cecum.

Epidemiology/Pathogenesis

- Sigmoid volvulus is seen in older patients with a history of constipation and redundant sigmoid colon.
- Cecal volvulus results in patients with congenitally anomalous fixation of the right colon but may also be seen secondary to adhesions and Hirschsprung disease.

Clinical Manifestations

- Sudden onset of abdominal pain, nausea, vomiting, and obstipation.

- Compromise in the vascular supply can result in strangulation, infarction, perforation, and peritonitis that present with fever, guarding, rigidity, and rebound.

Diagnosis

- Plain radiograph abdomen: In sigmoid volvulus, massively dilated sigmoid colon with proximal colonic dilatation is seen. The appearance of the sigmoid colon that can extend from the pelvis into the right upper quadrant resembles a bent inner tube or an omega. In patients with a cecal volvulus, the cecum is seen as a kidney-shaped mass in the left upper quadrant.
- CT scan of the abdomen is necessary to make a definitive diagnosis with a characteristic whirl pattern of the sigmoid colon around its mesentery and vascular supply with a bird beak appearance of the afferent and efferent bowel segments.

Treatment

- Cecal volvulus is treated with cecal resection, cecopexy, or cecostomy. Colonoscopy should not be performed due to the risk of perforation.
- Sigmoid volvulus can be treated with flexible sigmoidoscopy with resultant decompression of the sigmoid colon and placement of a rectal tube. Flexile sigmoidoscopy is contraindicated in patients with gangrene, perforation, or peritonitis. Surgery with resection and primary anastomosis or the Hartman procedure with a sigmoidopexy should be considered in patients to prevent recurrence.

Acute Colonic Pseudo-obstruction (Ogilvie's Syndrome)

Acute dilatation of the cecum and the right colon that occurs in the absence of an obstructing lesion or intrinsic disease of the colon.

Etiology/Pathogenesis

The etiology is unknown, but conditions associated with acute colonic pseudo-obstruction are orthopedic, pelvic, and abdominal surgery, trauma, heart failure, metabolic abnormalities, and serious infections.

Clinical Manifestations

- Massive abdominal distension is the predominant feature.
- Nausea, vomiting, abdominal pain, constipation, and, paradoxically, diarrhea may be seen.
- Perforation or ischemia is rare unless the diameter of the cecum is >12 cm.

Physical Examination

The abdomen is distended, tympanitic on percussion, and bowel sounds are frequently present but may be hypoactive or absent. The presence of guarding, rigidity, and rebound suggest impending perforation.

Diagnosis

- Laboratory tests: Electrolyte abnormalities (hypokalemia, hypocalcemia, hypomagnesemia), normal white blood cell count.
- The diagnosis is made on the basis of radiographs, and although there is no consensus, a cecal diameter of 9 cm is used as a cutoff. KUB (kidney, ureter, bladder) shows a dilated colon, often from the cecum to the splenic flexure, and occasionally to the rectum with normal haustral markings.
- CT scan or barium enema can definitively rule out a mechanical obstruction but should be performed only after perforation has been ruled out.

Differential Diagnosis

In patients with paralytic ileus-abdominal distention is less and radiographs show air fluid levels. In large bowel obstruction from a mechanical cause there is an abrupt cut off with the lack of gas in the distal colon or rectum. Patients with toxic megacolon have fever, severe abdominal pain, and radiographs show thumb printing due to submucosal edema.

Treatment

- Initial management of acute colonic pseudo-obstruction is conservative for the first 24 to 48 h provided the cecal diameter is <12 cm. This consists of the following:
  - Treatment of the underlying disease.
  - NPO.
  - Nasogastric and rectal decompression.
  - Intravenous fluids and correction of electrolyte abnormalities.
  - Discontinuance of medications that may decrease colonic motility (e.g., calcium channel blockers, anticholinergic agents, opioids)
  - Serial physical exams and radiographs every 12 h.
- Neostigmine: Studies have demonstrated that neostigmine, an acetylcholinesterase inhibitor, is effective in producing rapid colonic decompression. Side effects include transient crampy abdominal pain, salivation, vomiting, and symptomatic bradycardia; therefore, neostigmine should be administered cautiously while monitoring patients on telemetry.
- Colonoscopy: If symptoms persist or worsen despite neostigmine use, or if the colonic diameter increases or remains above

12 cm, colonoscopy is indicated for decompression. The risk of recurrence may be decreased by the placement of a drainage tube in the right colon at the time of colonoscopy.
- Surgery (cecostomy or colectomy) is indicated for patients who fail medical management and colonoscopic decompression; cecal diameter is >14 cm; or in cases of perforation.

MESENTERIC ISCHEMIA

Acute Mesenteric Ischemia

Acute mesenteric ischemia is a reduction in splanchnic blood flow secondary to arterial occlusion from thrombus, embolus, vasospasm, or venous occlusion.
- Arterial embolic disease: Usually involves the superior mesenteric artery (SMA). Risk factors include atrial fibrillation, recent myocardial infarction, valvular heart disease, and recent cardiac or vascular catheterization.
- Artery thrombosis: Occurs at areas of severe atherosclerotic narrowing, most commonly at the origin of the SMA. The acute ischemic episode is commonly seen in patients with symptoms of chronic ischemia with post-prandial abdominal pain.
- Nonocclusive mesenteric ischemia (NOMI): Occurs secondary to hypoperfusion as seen in cardiogenic, distributive, or hypovolemic shock.
- Venous thrombosis: Associated with the presence of a hypercoagulable state including malignancy, proteins C and S deficiency, antithrombin III deficiency, antiphospholipid antibody syndrome, pancreatitis, portal hypertension, and trauma.

Clinical Manifestations

- Abdominal pain with severe pain out of proportion to the physical exam. Small bowel ischemia pain is usually periumbilical. Pain is usually sudden in onset with embolic occlusion but may be gradual with thrombosis or vasospasm.
- Hematochezia is the passage of maroon or bright red blood per rectum, although characteristic of colonic ischemia, may be the only finding in acute mesenteric ischemia AMI.
- Diarrhea with increased bowel activity secondary to early ischemia may be seen in association with fever, nausea, and vomiting.

Physical Examination

- Initially unremarkable with minimal distension and hypoactive bowel sounds.
- Guarding, rigidity, and rebound suggest the presence of peritonitis.

Diagnosis

- Laboratory tests: Metabolic acidosis and elevated lactic acid develop suggest bowel necrosis.
- Abdominal radiograph
  - Nonspecific findings including the presence of an ileus with distended loops bowel
  - Thumb printing seen due to the presence of air within the bowel wall (pneumatosis intestinalis).
  - Portal venous gas
  - Air under the diaphragm with perforation
- CT angiography: Used to make a diagnosis and rule out other causes of acute abdominal pain.
- Angiography is the gold standard for the diagnosis and treatment of acute mesenteric ischemia. It should be performed early when this disorder is suspected.

Management

Initial management consists of the following:

- Hemodynamic monitoring with careful monitoring of volume status.
- Intravenous hydration and repletion of electrolytes.
- Discontinuation of vasoconstrictors.
- Anticoagulation with heparin in patients with mesenteric vein thrombosis unless there is active bleeding.
- Angiography is both diagnostic and therapeutic as are embolectomy, thrombolysis, thrombectomy, the use of vasodilators in patients with NOMI, or it provides important information for an arterial bypass. With such procedures, bowel that initially appears infarcted may show surprising recovery after blood flow is restored.
- Short segments of bowel that are nonviable or of questionable viability after revascularization are resected, and a primary anastomosis is performed. If extensive portions of bowel are of questionable viability, necrotic bowel is resected and a second-look laparotomy is performed within 12 to 24 h to demarcate viable and nonviable bowel in order to minimize resection (Fig. 5-3).

Chronic Mesenteric Ischemia

Epidemiology/Pathogenesis

Chronic mesenteric ischemia (CMI) results from atherosclerotic narrowing of the splanchnic vessels with obstruction of at least two of the three major splanchnic arteries before symptoms of ischemia manifest. CMI may be secondary to insufficient blood supply to meet an increase in demand after a meal or increased demand for

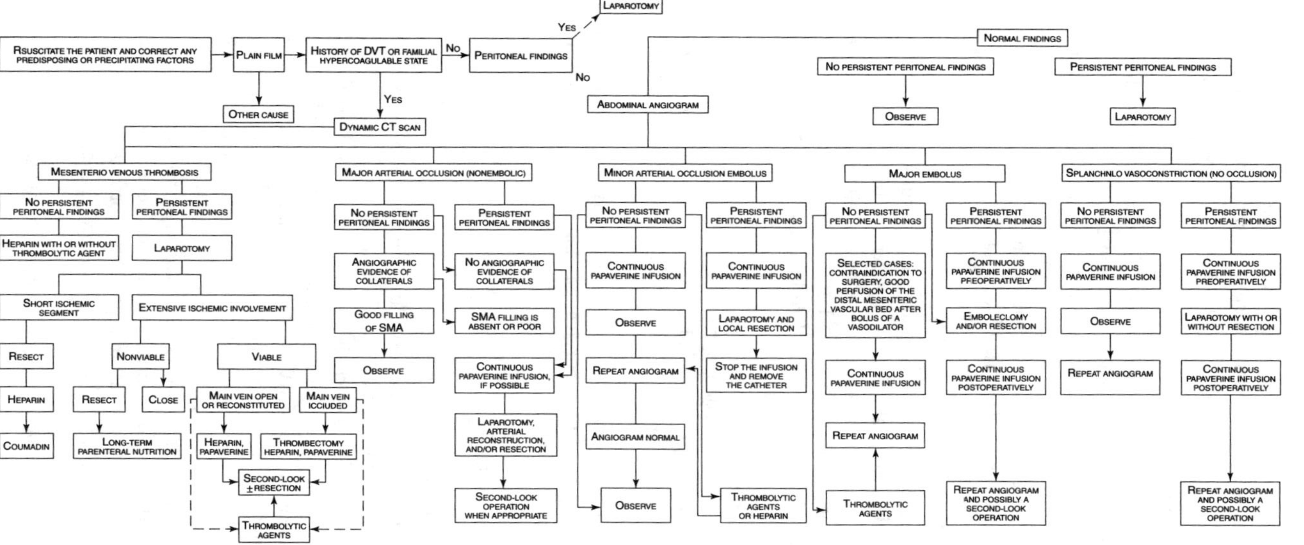

Figure 5-3 • Algorithm for the diagnosis and treatment of acute intestinal ischemia. Solid lines indicate accepted management plans and dashed lines indicate alternate management plans. SMA, superior mesenteric artery; DVT, deep vein thrombosis. (From American Gastroenterological Association Medical position statement: guidelines on intestinal ischemia. *Gastroenterology.* 2000;118:951, with permission.)

gastric blood flow as food enters the stomach. The presence of food in the stomach results in a steal of blood supply from the small intestine to the stomach and manifests as abdominal pain.

Clinical Manifestations

- Abdominal pain that characteristically occurs within the first hour after a large meal and subsides in 1 to 2 h.
- Asymptomatic, until acute mesenteric ischemia results from thrombus formation, at which time patients present with sudden onset of severe abdominal pain.
- Weight loss due to decreased food intake.

Diagnosis

- Mesenteric duplex ultrasonography is a useful screening test for high-grade stenosis and is used in patients with renal failure who cannot undergo angiography. In patients with positive duplex, angiography must be performed prior to revascularization.
- Angiography is the gold standard in diagnosing CMI.

Treatment

- Surgical revascularization: Bypass surgery, mesenteric endarterectomy, and reimplantation of the SMA can be performed in patients who are good surgical candidates, have typical symptoms and positive angiography.
- Percutaneous transluminal angioplasty is an alternative in patients who are poor surgical candidates and in whom the diagnosis is uncertain.

Colonic Ischemia

Epidemiology/Pathogenesis

- Ischemic colitis is the most frequent form of mesenteric ischemia, affecting mostly elderly individuals.
- It occurs secondary to occlusive or nonocclusive disease of the inferior mesenteric artery (IMA), colonic branches of the SMA, superior mesenteric vein (SMV), and inferior mesenteric vein (IMV).
- Ischemic colitis predominantly affects the left colon, specifically the watershed areas of the splenic flexure and rectosigmoid junction, but spares the rectum.
- It includes a spectrum of disorders according to the ischemic injury:
  - Acute transient self-limited ischemia (reversible colopathy with mucosal as well as submucosal hemorrhage)
  - Acute fulminant ischemia (transmural ischemia that progresses to necrosis)
  - Chronic ischemic colitis (partially reversible and manifests as colonic stenosis)

Clinical Manifestations

Ischemic colitis often occurs with no clear identifiable precipitant.

- Sudden onset of crampy left lower quadrant abdominal pain.
- Diarrhea with the passage of bright red blood within 24 h of onset
- Nausea, vomiting, abdominal distension may be seen

Physical Examination

Tachycardia, low-grade fever, reveals only mild to moderate abdominal tenderness over the involved segment of bowel, fecal occult blood positive. Guarding, rigidity, or rebound tenderness suggest bowel gangrene and perforation.

Differential Diagnosis

Infectious colitis, IBD, radiation colitis, diverticulitis

Diagnosis

- Stool studies for fecal leukocytes, ova, and parasites, *Clostridium difficile* toxin, and stool cultures for *Salmonella*, *Shigella*, *Campylobacter*, and *Escherichia coli* 0157:H7 are necessary to exclude infectious colitis.
- Plain films are nonspecific but may reveal thumb printing due to bowel wall edema. Pneumatosis intestinalis (gas in the bowel wall) or the portal vein suggests bowel infarction.
- Colonoscopy with biopsy is the test of choice. In ischemic colitis the mucosa is edematous, hemorrhagic, friable, and ulcerated. Biopsy shows congested mucosa, submucosal hemorrhage, inflammatory infiltrate, and loss of superficial cells. Hemosiderin deposition with fibrosis is seen with chronic disease.
- Abdominal CT scan is not necessary to make a diagnosis of ischemic colitis but helps to rule out other causes of abdominal pain. Mesenteric angiography is usually not indicated in the management of colonic ischemia, as colonic blood flow has usually returned to normal by the time of presentation.

Treatment

Initial treatment is supportive

- NPO.
- Intravenous hydration and repletion of electrolyte abnormalities.
- Serial physical examination.
- Broad-spectrum antibiotics.
- Avoid/discontinue vasoconstrictors.
- If the patient improves: Colonoscopy can be repeated at 1 to 2 weeks, segmental colitis on colonoscopy, stricture formation, recurrent fever, or sepsis should all be treated with resection.

- If the patient develops fever, leukocytosis, continued diarrhea, or bleeding despite conservative management, or if peritoneal signs develop, laparotomy and segment resection of the bowel are indicated.
- Surgery is also indicated in patients with protein-losing enteropathy from persistent ischemic lesions, recurrent sepsis, and long-term complications such as stenosis.

Prognosis

The majority of patients (85%) with ischemia have a self-limited course, and a minority develops long-term complications such as persistent segmental colitis and strictures.

Diverticular Disease

Diverticula of the colon are outpouchings of the mucosa and submucosa through a defect in the muscular layer of the intestine. This herniation occurs at the site of penetration of the vasa recta through the circular muscle between the tenia coli (Fig. 5-4).

- The exact etiology is unknown but may be due to increased intraluminal pressure seen in patients on low-fiber diets with constipation.
- Prevalence of diverticulosis increases with age.
- Diverticula are most commonly seen in the colon and are predominantly in the sigmoid colon (Fig. 5-5).

Clinical Manifestations

- Most patients with diverticulosis are asymptomatic and diagnosis is incidental on barium enema or colonoscopy obtained for some other indication.
- Even in the absence of infection, diverticulosis can be associated with intermittent crampy left lower quadrant pain and may be associated with alterations in bowel habits.
- Fever and leukocytosis are characteristically absent.
- Physical examination reveals only mild tenderness in the left lower quadrant with no peritoneal signs.

Diagnosis

- Abdominal CT scan with oral contrast can visualize diverticula, but inflammation is characteristically absent. In addition the scan helps to exclude other causes of abdominal pain.
- Flexible sigmoidoscopy and colonoscopy are relatively contraindicated if diverticulitis is suspected but enable visualization of wide-mouth diverticulae.

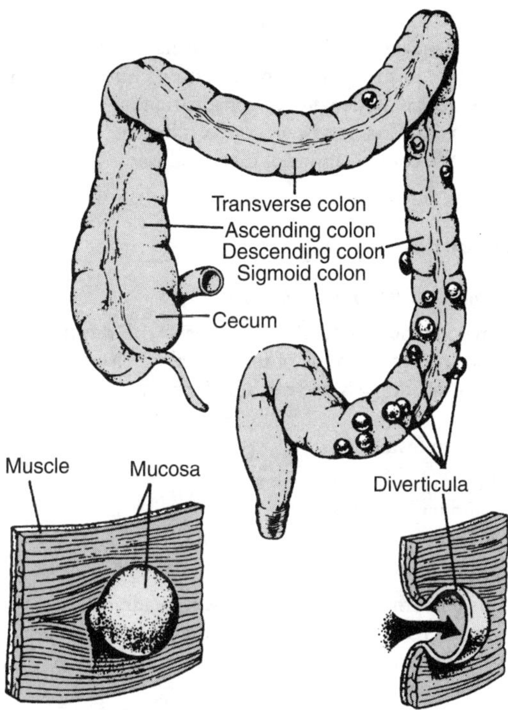

Figure 5-4 • Diverticula are most common in the sigmoid colon; they diminish in number and size as the colon approaches the cecum. Diverticula are rarely found in the rectum.

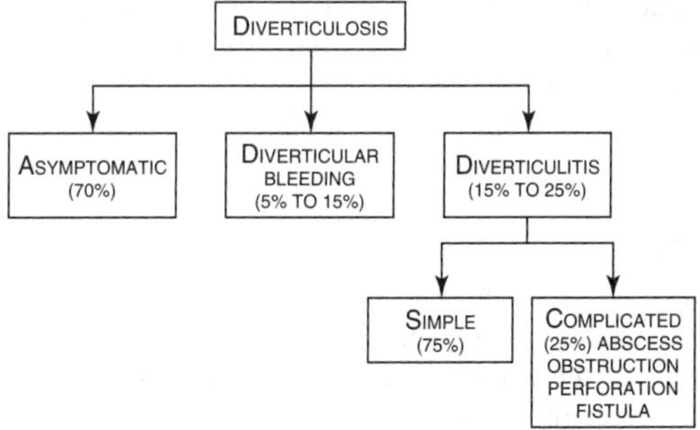

Figure 5-5 • Natural history of diverticulosis. (Reproduced with permission from Young-Fadok T and Pemberton J. *Clinical Manifestations and Diagnosis of Colonic Diverticular Disease*. In:UpToDate, Rose, BD (Ed), UpToDate, Waltham, MA, 2006. Copyright 2006 UpToDate, Inc. For more information visit www.uptodate.com)

Treatment

- Medical management: High-fiber diets have not been shown to be effective in preventing complications but are of symptomatic benefit in patients with constipation.
- Avoidance of nuts, seeds, or popcorn has not been shown to decrease the complications of diverticulosis.

Diverticulitis

Epidemiology/Pathogenesis

It is estimated that 15% to 20% of patients with diverticulosis will develop diverticulitis. Erosion of the wall of the diverticulum results in inflammation, necrosis, and microperforation.

Clinical Manifestations

- Left lower quadrant abdominal pain
- Fever and leukocytosis

Physical Examination

- Reveals tenderness over the left lower quadrant
- Guarding, rigidity, and rebound indicate the development of peritonitis from a presumed perforation.

Complications

Perforation, obstruction, abscess, or fistula

Diagnosis

- CT abdomen: The presence of sigmoid diverticula; thickened colonic wall >4 mm; inflammation within the pericolic fat; the collection of contrast material or fluid.
- Barium enema or colonoscopy should not be performed due to the high risk of perforation.

Treatment

- Simple diverticulitis: Treat conservatively.
  - Diet: NPO until the pain resolves.
  - Antibiotic therapy: With a fluoroquinolone and metronidazole.
- Complicated diverticulitis:
  - Complications including peritonitis, persistent obstruction, abscess not amenable to percutaneous drainage, failure of conservative management or fistula require operative intervention.
  - Other indications for surgery are the inability to exclude a malignancy and recurrent episodes of diverticulitis.

Colorectal Cancer

Epidemiology/Pathogenesis

- Colorectal cancer (CRC) is the second leading cause of cancer death in the United States. The lifetime incidence of CRC in patients at average risk is about 5%, with 90% of cases occurring after age 50 (Fig. 5-6).
- Analysis of colorectal adenomas and carcinomas at the molecular level has led to the genetic model of colon carcinogenesis in which cancer develops as a result of accumulation of multiple genetic alterations (Kinzler KW, Vogelstein B. Colorectal tumors. In: Vogelstein B, Kinzler KW, eds. *The genetic basis of human cancer*. New York: McGraw-Hill; 1998:565–587).

Risk Factors

- Personal history of colon cancer or colon polyps.
- Individuals with inherited conditions such as hereditary nonpolyposis colorectal cancer (HNPCC) and familial adenomatous polyposis (FAP) have a close to 80% to 100% risk of developing CRC, in addition to extraintestinal cancers in patients with HNPCC.
- Inflammatory bowel disease: Incidence of colon cancer increases 8 to 10 years after the onset of ulcerative colitis in those patients with disease beyond the splenic flexure with an increase of 0.5% per year between 10 and 20 years and 1% per year thereafter.
- Smoking: Studies have shown an increased incidence and mortality from colon cancer in cigarette smokers.
- Alcohol consumption.
- Cholecystectomy has been associated with an increased risk for right-sided colon cancers.
- Diabetes: Hyperinsulinemia in diabetes and insulin therapy.

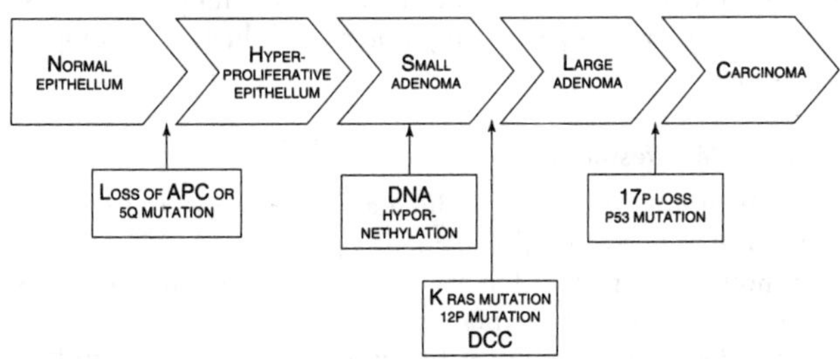

Figure 5-6 • Colon carcinogenesis is a multistep process resulting from well-defined genetic events. (Modified from Faeron ER, Vogelstein BA. *Cell*. 1990;61:759–767, with permission.)

Protective Factors

- Folate: May be beneficial in patients who are genetically predisposed.
- Calcium: Observational studies have associated increased intake of calcium and vitamin D with a decreased risk of colorectal cancer and recurrent polyps. It is proposed that calcium acts early in the pathway of carcinogenesis, and a randomized trial by Baron et al. that found that calcium supplementation caused a moderate but statistically significant reduction in recurrent adenomas. However, a randomized, double-blind, placebo-controlled trial by Wactawski-Wende et al. (*N Engl J Med.* 2006;354:684–696) involved 36,282 postmenopausal women of which 18,176 women received 500 mg of elemental calcium as calcium carbonate with 200 IU of vitamin D_3 twice daily. Supplementation for 7 years had no effect on the incidence of colorectal cancer. However, the null finding may be related to the long latency associated with the development of colorectal cancer.
- Aspirin and nonsteroidal anti-inflammatory drugs (NSAIDs): The exact mechanism by which NSAIDs decrease the risk of colon cancer is unclear but may be secondary to the inhibition of COX-2 and increased apoptosis.
- Hormone replacement therapy (HRT): The national Polyprevention trial found no overall decrease in risk of adenoma recurrence in patients on HRT.

Pathology

- The predominant histologic subtype is adenocarcinoma; other subtypes are mucinous, signet ring cell carcinoma, squamous, adenosquamous, small cell, and undifferentiated.
- Adenocarcinoma of the colon arises from adenomatous polyps.
- Adenomas are divided into tubular, villous, and tubulovillous.
- Risk factors for development of cancer are villous adenomas, increasing polyps size (>1 cm), polyps with high-grade dysplasia, and cancer.

Clinical Manifestations

- Small tumors may not produce any symptoms and may be discovered incidentally on colonoscopy.
- Tumors in the right colon are polypoid masses and present as occult bleeding and anemia.
- Left colon tumors are obstructive apple core lesions and result in change in stool caliber, constipation, and tenesmus.
- Abdominal pain may occur secondary to bowel obstruction, perforation, peritonitis or peritoneal dissemination.

- Patients often have iron deficiency anemia; rectal cancer presents with hematochezia.
- Fever and weight loss.
- Metastatic disease: Dissemination to the liver, lung, brain, and bone.
- *Streptococcus bovis* and *Clostridium septicum* bacteremia may be the presenting feature.

Physical Examination

- Supraclavicular adenopathy
- Periumbilical nodule (Sister Mary Joseph)
- Colonic masses rarely palpable
- Hepatomegaly from metastatic disease
- Hemoccult positive stool

Diagnosis

- Colonoscopy is the test of choice as it allows lesions to be directly visualized and biopsied.
- Barium enema or virtual colonoscopy should be performed if full colonoscopy cannot be performed, because of an obstructing lesion, in order to determine if synchronous lesions are present more proximally.

Staging

- Table 5-3 presents the TNM (tumor, nodes, metastases) staging for colorectal cancer.
- CT abdomen and pelvis: Should be performed to determine tumor size, lymph nodes, and distant metastasis.
- Positron emission tomography (PET) scan: Indicated preoperatively in patients thought to have isolated liver lesions and in patients with rising carcinoembryonic antigen (CEA) levels and nondiagnostic CT scans.
- Endoscopic ultrasound (EUS): Indicated to determine depth of tumor invasion in patients with rectal cancer.
- CEA: Should not be used as a screening tool, but is used in patients with diagnosed colon cancer preoperatively to assess prognosis and disease recurrence.

Treatment

- Surgery
  - Lesions of the right colon, cecum, ascending colon, hepatic flexure or transverse colon are treated with right hemicolectomy with dissection of lymph nodes.
  - Lesions of the splenic flexure to the sigmoid colon are treated with left hemicolectomy and primary anastomosis to the rectum.
  - Lesions of the sigmoid are treated with a low anterior resection.
  - Lesions of the rectosigmoid resection and colostomy are needed.

TABLE 5-3 TNM Staging for Colorectal Cancer

Primary Tumor (T)
TX Primary tumor cannot be assessed
T0 No evidence of primary tumor
Tis Carcinoma *in situ:* intraepithelial or invasion of lamina propria[a]
T1 Tumor invades submucosa
T2 Tumor invades muscularis propria
T3 Tumor invades through the muscularis propria into the subserosa, or into nonperitonealized pericolic or perirectal tissues
T4 Tumor directly invades other organs or structures, and/or perforates visceral peritoneum[b,c]

Regional Lymph Nodes (N)
NX Regional lymph nodes cannot be assessed
N0 No regional lymph node metastasis
N1 Metastasis in 1 to 3 regional lymph nodes
N2 Metastasis in four or more regional lymph nodes

Distant Metastasis (M)
MX Distant metastasis cannot be assessed
M0 No distant metastasis
M1 Distant metastasis

[a]*Tis includes cancer cells confined within the glandular basement membrane (intraepithelial) or lamina propria (intramuscular) with no extension through the muscularis mucosae into the submucosa.*
[b]*Direct invasion in T4 includes invasion of other segments of the colorectum by way of the serosa; for example, invasion of the sigmoid colon by a carcinoma of the cecum.*
[c]*Tumor that is adherent to other organs or structures, macroscopically, is classified T4. However, if no tumor is present in the adhesion, microscopically, the classification should be pT3. The V and L substaging should be used to identify the presence or absence of vascular or lymphatic invasion.*

From American Joint Committee on Cancer (AJCC), *Staging manual. 6th ed.* New York: Springer-Verlag; 2002, with permission.

- Chemotherapy: Adjuvant chemotherapy (chemotherapy in patients who have undergone surgical resection with the intent to cure) in patients with Stage III colon cancer. Chemotherapy regimes include 5-fluorouracil (5-FU)/levamisole, capecitabine, and oxaliplatin.
- Postoperative surveillance: Colonoscopy should be performed preoperatively; however, if not performed should be done between 3 and 6 months postoperatively. If the preoperative or postoperative colonoscopy is normal, the next colonoscopy should be performed at 3 years, and then if normal every 5 years.
- Radiotherapy (RT): Studies have demonstrated a significant benefit to radiotherapy alone and an additional benefit when postoperative RT is combined with 5-FU-based regimens in patients with Stage II and Stage III rectal cancer.

TABLE 5-4 Five Year Survival for Colon Cancer According to Stage

Stage I (T1–2N0)	93%
Stage IIA (T3N0)	85%
Stage IIB (T4N0)	72%
Stage IIIA (T1–2N1)	83%
Stage IIIB (T3–4N1)	64%
Stage IIIC (N2)	44%
Stage IV	8%

From O'Connell JB, *J Natl Cancer Inst*. 2004 Oct 6;96(19):1420–1425, with permission.

Prognosis

- Table 5-4 presents the 5-year survival for colon cancer according to stage..

Chapter

6 Diseases of the Liver

ABNORMAL LIVER FUNCTION TESTS

- Liver function tests (LFT) if abnormal must always be confirmed.
- Elevations that are above twice the normal value must be interpreted in context of the clinical presentation of an individual patient.
- Important history in evaluation of abnormal liver function tests includes the following:
  - Alcohol
  - Medication/Drugs
  - Family history of liver disease: Wilson's disease, alpha-1-antitrypsin deficiency, hemochromatosis, celiac sprue, inherited disorders of muscle metabolism

Exercise

- Further evaluation of the abnormal LFTs depends on the pattern of elevation:
  - Elevated transaminases
  - Elevated alkaline phosphatase
  - Elevated bilirubin
  - Elevated PT (prothrombin time) and low albumin

Elevated Transaminases

- Alanine aminotransferase (ALT) is predominantly derived from the hepatocyte; however, aspartate transaminases (AST) is derived from hepatocyte mitochondria and cytosol, as well as skeletal muscle, heart, lungs, pancreas, brain, and leukocytes.
- Elevation of both AST and ALT reflect hepatocyte damage and necrosis.
- Degree of elevation does not correspond to the extent of necrosis or prognosis.
- Transaminases greater than 15 times the upper limit are seen with viral hepatitis, drug ingestion (acetaminophen), shock liver, and fulminant Wilson's disease.
- Causes of mild to moderate elevation in transaminases are listed in Table 6-1.
- Pattern of transaminase elevation may provide a clue to the etiology with AST > ALT in alcohol-induced liver injury. This pattern is secondary to the following:

TABLE 6-1 Causes of Mild Increases in ALT and AST

Hepatic: Predominantly ALT
Chronic hepatitis C
Chronic hepatitis B
Acute viral hepatitis (A–E, EBV, CMV)
Steatosis/steatohepatitis
Hemachromatosis
Medications/toxins
Autoimmune hepatitis
alpha-1-Antitrypsin deficiency
Wilson's disease
Celiac sprue
Hepatic: Predominantly AST
Alcohol-related liver injury
Steatosis/steatohepatitis
Cirrhosis
Nonhepatic
Hemolysis
Myopathy
Thyroid disease
Strenuous exercise

From Richard M Green, Steven Flomin. AGA Technical review on the evaluation of liver chemistry tests. *Gastroenterology* 123, 2002;1364–1384.

- Deficiency in pyridoxal 5′-phosphate a cofactor for ALT and AST results in a greater decrease in ALT concentration.
- Mitochondrial injury secondary to alcohol with release of AST.

• Further workup of elevated transaminases is outlined in Figure 6-1.

Elevated Alkaline Phosphatase

• Alkaline phosphatase is derived from the biliary tract, liver, intestine, kidney, and the placenta.
• Alkaline phosphatase elevation results from synthesis following injury and not release from damaged tissue. Patients with injury to the biliary tree may therefore have elevated transaminases before an increase in alkaline phosphatase.
• The first step in the evaluation of an elevated alkaline phosphatase is to determine if it is hepatobiliary in origin by checking levels of gamma glutamyl transpeptidase (GGT). GGT is sensitive but not specific for hepatobiliary disease. Elevation of GGT and alkaline phosphatase suggests a hepatobiliary process (Fig. 6-2).

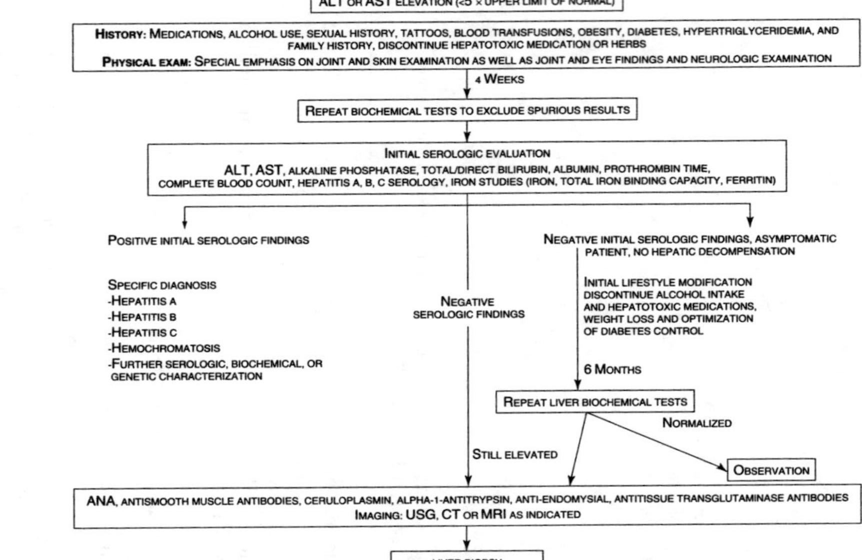

Figure 6-1 • Increased liver function tests in an asymptomatic patient. (Modified and reprinted from R. Green and S. Flamm, AGA medical position statement and technical review on the evaluation of liver chemistry tests, Gastroenterology, 2002;123:1364–1384. Goseling W, Friedman L. *Clin Gastroenterol Hepatol.* 2005;3(9):835, Figure 2, with permission.)

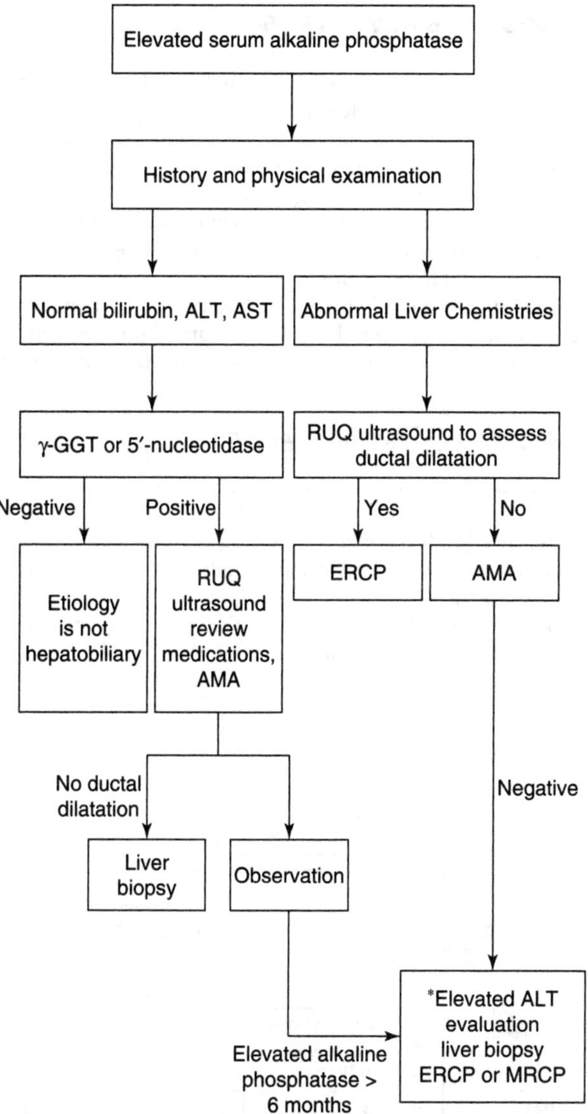

Figure 6-2 • Diagnosing the patient with elevated serum alkaline phosphatase (AP) levels. CT, computed tomography; ERCP, endoscopic retrograde cholangiopancreatography; GGT, serum γ-glutamyltransferase; 5′NT, 5′-nucleotidase. (Reprinted from Gastroenterology V123(4) American *Gastroenterological Association medical position statement: Evaluation of liver chemistry tests*, 1364–1366; 2002 with permission of the American Gastroenterological Association.)

HYPERBILIRUBINEMIA (FIG. 6-3)

- Elevated bilirubin must be fractionated to determine if direct or indirect bilirubin is elevated.
- Conjugated hyperbilirubinemia: Defined as a conjugated bilirubin >30% of the total bilirubin.
- Unconjugated bilirubin is tightly bound to albumin and not excreted by the kidneys. In contrast, conjugated bilirubin is not tightly bound to albumin, is therefore excreted by the kidneys, and is detectable in the urine.
- An elevation in direct bilirubin (conjugated) implies that there is decreased excretion into bile canaliculi after bilirubin is conjugated secondary to liver disease or obstruction of the bile ducts.

Unconjugated Hyperbilirubinemia

- Elevation of indirect bilirubin (unconjugated) results from the following:
  - Increased production: Intravascular or extravascular hemolysis. Typically never elevated >5 mg/dL unless there is concomitant liver disease
  - Decreased uptake of bilirubin by the liver: Congestive heart failure and portocaval shunts due to decreased blood flow to the liver

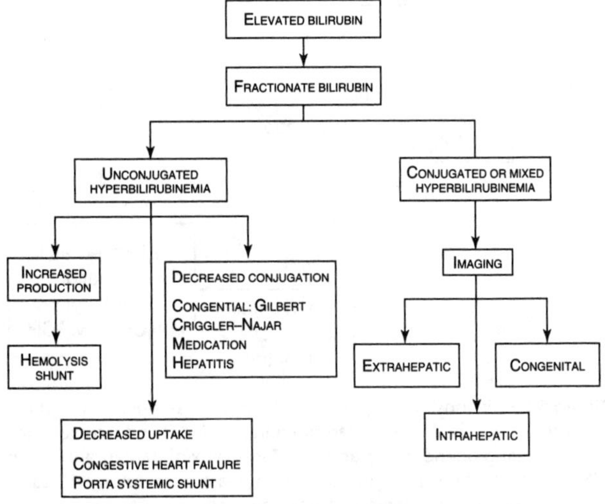

Figure 6-3 • Elevated bilirubin.

- Defect in conjugation: Medications, e.g. Nonsteroidal anti-inflammatory drugs (NSAIDs), rifampin; Gilbert's syndrome and Crigler–Najar, hepatitis (hepatitis A to E, cytomegalovirus, Epstein–Barr virus).

Conjugated Hyperbilirubinemia

Congenital Conjugated Hyperbilirubinemias

- *Rotor syndrome*: An autosomal recessive, asymptomatic disorder characterized by mixed hyperbilirubinemia secondary to defective excretion of bilirubin. Total bilirubin levels rarely exceed 5 mg/dL and increase with physical stress and infection. Other LFTs are characteristically normal.
- *Dubin–Johnson syndrome*: Autosomal recessive disorder that results from defective ATP-mediated transport of bilirubin glucoronide. Similar to Rotor syndrome, patients have mixed or conjugated hyperbilirubinemia, normal liver function tests, and elevated urine coproporphyrin. Liver biopsy specimens have characteristic darkly pigmented liver.
- Both Dubin–Johnson and Rotor syndromes are asymptomatic but important to diagnose to avoid repetitive testing in patients who have mixed hyperbilirubinemia.

Extrahepatic Cholestasis

Obstruction of the bile ducts results in the mixed hyperbilirubinemia as conjugated bilirubin in hepatocytes undergoes deconjugation. In addition to bilirubin, bile salts and pigments are transported into the plasma. Patients with biliary obstruction therefore have elevated conjugated and unconjugated bilirubin, urine bilirubin, and elevated alkaline phosphatase from injury to the bile duct.

Intrahepatic Cholestasis

- Disorders that can cause intrahepatic cholestasis include primary biliary cirrhosis, primary sclerosing cholangitis, hepatitis, sepsis, medications, total parenteral nutrition (TPN), and pregnancy. It is, however, important to note that these conditions may also cause an elevation in alkaline phosphatase as do extrahepatic causes of biliary obstruction; imaging is indicated to determine the etiology.
- Imaging studies to differentiate intrahepatic from extrahepatic causes of cholestasis:
  - Right upper quadrant ultrasound (USG): Can be used to detect stones in the gallbladder (cholelithiasis), stones in the bile duct (choledocholithiasis), and extrahepatic biliary ductal dilatation. The advantage of USG is that it is widely

available and inexpensive; however, the sensitivity is operator dependent (50% to 90% sensitive) and stones in the common bile duct (CBD) may not be visualized due to bowel gas.

- Abdominal computed tomography (CT): Can detect intrahepatic and extrahepatic ductal dilatation and has the advantage of visualizing the rest the abdomen/pelvis. Noncalcified stones that are seen on USG may be missed on CT scans, which are also a more expensive diagnostic modality.
- Endoscopic retrograde cholangiopancreatography (ERCP): The main advantage of an ERCP is that it is both diagnostic and therapeutic. It allows for direct visualization of the biliary and pancreatic ducts, allows for therapeutic interventions such as stone extraction, papillotomy, and stent placement.
- Magnetic resonance cholangiopancreatography (MRCP): MRCP is 90% to 100% sensitive in detecting biliary ductal dilatation and the level of obstruction. The disadvantage of a MRCP is its expense as a diagnostic modality and the lack of therapeutic benefit.
- Percutaneous transhepatic cholangiogram (PTC): PTC involves the injection of contrast medium percutaneously through a catheter inserted into the hepatic parenchyma and advanced into the biliary tree. PTC is indicated in patients with intrahepatic duct obstruction or in cases where ERCP is contraindicated.

- Albumin and PT are the most sensitive indicators of acute hepatic dysfunction since both are predominantly synthesized in the liver.

ACUTE HEPATITIS

- Hepatitis is a nonspecific term that refers to hepatocellular injury and necrosis.
- Hepatitis is defined as acute if the inflammatory response lasts for less than 6 months and chronic if the duration of inflammation is greater than 6 months.

Hepatitis A

Epidemiology/Pathogenesis

- Hepatitis A virus (HAV) is an RNA virus in the Hepadnavirus genus of the Picornaviridae that causes acute hepatitis.
- HAV is spread by the feco-oral route and is commonly seen in conditions of poor sanitation.
- Incubation period of HAV ranges from 2 to 6 weeks.

Clinical Manifestations

- Clinical manifestations vary with age.
- Children frequently have an acute and often subclinical illness.
- Adults are frequently symptomatic and symptoms are similar to all other forms of hepatitis with fatigue, malaise, nausea, vomiting, jaundice, dark urine, and clay-colored stool.
- In rare cases ((0.5%), adults present with fulminant hepatic failure with signs of hepatic failure and encephalopathy.

Physical Examination

- Icterus
- Tender hepatomegaly
- Occasional splenomegaly

Diagnosis

- Liver function tests
  - Elevated transaminases (ALT > AST ~ 1000 IU/L) precede the onset of clinical features by 1 to 2 weeks and resolve in 4 to 5 weeks.
  - Total bilirubin peaks following peak in transaminases.
- Serology (Fig. 6-4)
  - Anti-HAV immunoglobulin M (IgM) is produced at the onset of symptoms and peaks in the convalescent phase. In a patient with symptoms a positive HAV IgM is diagnostic of acute infection.

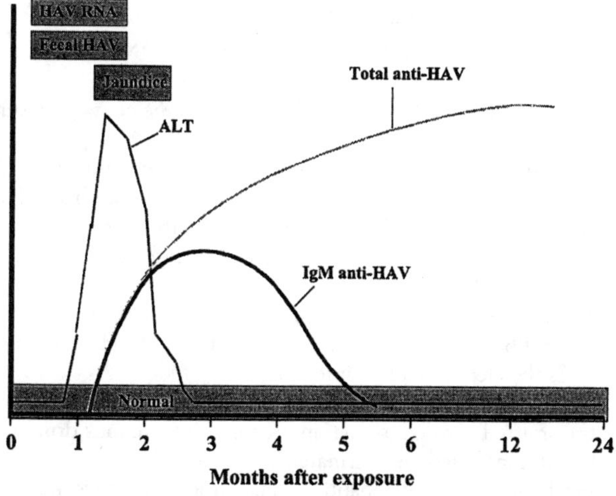

Figure 6-4 • Typical serologic course of acute hepatitis A virus infection. (From Yamada T, Alpers D, Kaplowitz N, et al. *Textbook of gastroenterology*. Vol. 2. 4th ed. Baltimore: Lippincott Williams & Wilkins; 2003:2290, with permission.)

- However, anti-HAV IgM persists for 4 to 6 weeks and may therefore indicate past infection and should be interpreted with caution.
- Anti-HAV IgG appears early in the convalescent phase of the disease, and remains detectable for decades.

Treatment

- Supportive care: Acute hepatitis A is a largely self-limited illness and resolves in 2 to 4 weeks.
- Patients with fulminant hepatitis need hospitalization and should be considered for liver transplantation.
- Prevention of HAV is possible with handwashing. Pre-exposure prophylaxis with hepatitis A immune globulin; confers immunity for 6 months. However immune globulin carries the risk of transmitting infection and is therefore reserved for patients with allergies to the hepatitis A vaccine or as part of postexposure prophylaxis.
- Hepatitis A vaccine is a formalin-inactivated vaccine. Indications for administration include travel to endemic areas and patients with chronic liver disease. It should be considered in high-risk groups such as patients receiving clotting factors, men who have sex with men (MSM), and drug users.

Hepatitis B

Epidemiology/Pathogenesis

- Hepatitis B virus (HBV) is a double-stranded DNA virus of the Hepadnavirus family.
- Hepatitis B virus is surrounded by an envelope containing surface antigen HBs Ag.
- The nucleocapsid contains the hepatitis B core antigen (HBc Ag) which unlike HBs Ag is not detectable in the serum. The antibody to hepatitis B core antigen (anti-Hbc) is detectable.
- Hepatitis Be antigen (HBe Ag) is an indicator of active viral replication.
- The presence of HBe Ag and HBV DNA indicate active viral replication whereas the presence of antibody to HBe Ag indicates the clearance of an infection.
- HBV is spread by the blood and body fluids. It is therefore transmitted through sexual intercourse, intravenous drug use, blood transfusion and perinatally.
- Incubation period of hepatitis B ranges from 2 to 24 weeks.
- Presentation of hepatitis B varies in the patients with acute hepatitis, chronic hepatitis, fulminant hepatitis, and an asymptomatic carrier state.

Clinical Manifestations

- Clinical manifestations are similar to all other forms of hepatitis with fatigue, malaise, nausea, vomiting, jaundice, right upper quadrant pain, dark urine, and clay-colored stool.
- Some patients may present with serum sickness-like illness with arthritis and rash.
- In rare cases (<1%), adults present with fulminant hepatic failure with signs of hepatic failure and encephalopathy.

Physical Examination

- Icterus
- Tender hepatomegaly
- Occasional splenomegaly

Diagnosis

- Liver function tests
  - Elevated transaminases (ALT > AST ~ 1000 IU/L) precede the onset of clinical features by 1 to 2 weeks and resolve in 4 to 12 weeks.
  - Persistent elevation of transaminases >6 months indicates the development of chronic hepatitis.
- Serology (Fig. 6-5)
  - Viral markers in acute infection: HBs Ag is the first marker of acute hepatitis B infection and persists for 1 to 2 months in an acute infection.

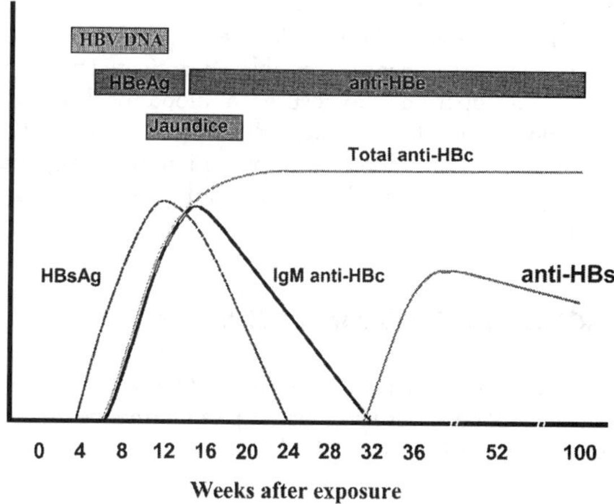

Figure 6-5 • Typical serologic course of acute hepatitis B virus infection. (From Yamada T, Alpers D, Kaplowitz N, et al. *Textbook of gastroenterology*. Vol. 2. 4th ed. Baltimore: Lippincott Williams & Wilkins; 2003:2290, with permission.)

- The presence of HBs Ag for >6 months indicates a chronic infection.
- Following the disappearance of HBs Ag and before the appearance of anti-HBs antibody, the antibody to core antigen (anti-HBc antibody) may the only marker in this window period.
- Anti-HBc antibody is not protective and only indicates exposure to hepatitis B.
- Anti-HBc antibody is initially IgM, with IgG produced later in the disease. IgM can therefore be used to distinguish acute from chronic infection. The presence of HBV DNA, HBe Ag in the absence of antibodies indicates the presence of an acute infection and active viral replication.
- Anti-HBe antibody is produced once HBe antigen has been cleared and indicates the absence of viral replication.

Treatment/Prognosis

- Supportive care
- Prognosis depends on the timing of infection. If acute infection occurs in childhood, 90% develop chronic hepatitis B; however, patients who are infected as adults often have an aggressive immune response and <10% develop chronic hepatitis B.
- HBV infection is a risk factor for hepatocellular carcinoma, which arises almost exclusively in patients with cirrhosis.
- Universal immunization is recommended for all newborns in the United States. Neonates of HBs Ag-positive mothers should receive hepatitis B immune globulin (HBIG) and hepatitis B vaccine simultaneously at birth.
- Postexposure prophylaxis includes the initiation of the hepatitis B vaccine series to any susceptible, unvaccinated person who sustains occupational exposure to blood or body fluid. Postexposure prophylaxis with HBIG and/or hepatitis B vaccine should be considered after evaluation of the hepatitis B surface antigen status of the source and the vaccination history and antibody status of the exposed person.

CHRONIC HEPATITIS B INFECTION

Chronic hepatitis B is defined by the presence of serum HBs Ag for more than 6 months. Chronic hepatitis B can further be subdivided on the basis of persistence of HBe Ag.

Inactive Carrier

An inactive hepatitis B carrier is defined as one with HBs Ag in the serum for greater than 6 months but without HBe Ag, with normal liver function tests, and with low levels of HBV DNA (<100,000 copies/mL). These patients remain at risk for hepatocellular carcinoma.

Precore Mutant

Hepatitis B virus has six possible genotypes, A through G. Predominant genotypes vary with demography as do the clinical features associated with hepatitis infection with each genotype. Patients with genotype A present as HBe Ag positive, whereas patients with genotypes other than genotype A frequently have HBe Ag negative chronic hepatitis. These individuals are infected with the hepatitis B with G1896 stop codon precore mutation that prevents the translation of a precore protein and therefore HBe antigen production. These individuals are HBs Ag positive, HBe Ag negative, anti-HBe antibody positive with detectable HBV DNA. Hepatitis B precore mutants are predominantly seen in the Mediterranean population. Persistently elevated or fluctuating levels of transaminases characterize the clinical course of patients with HBe Ag-negative hepatitis. Because the aim of treatment is to result in hepatitis Be antigen seroconversion, which by definition cannot be induced in these patients, treatment is continued indefinitely.

Reactivation

Reactivation of inactive carriers of hepatitis B or patients with resolved infection is characterized by elevation of liver function tests and the presence of HBe Ag and an elevation of HBV DNA.

Resolved Infection

Patients with past acute or chronic hepatitis who become HBs Ag negative, have no HBV DNA and normal liver function tests, and are anti-HBc and anti-HBs antibody positive. These patients remain at risk for disease reactivation when treated with immunosuppressive medication and in rare cases can transmit hepatitis B.

Phases of Chronic Hepatitis B Infection

- Replicative
  - Immune tolerance: Patients with perinatally acquired hepatitis B are HBe Ag positive and have high levels of HBV DNA but normal liver function tests and liver biopsy due to immune tolerance to hepatitis B. This phase of immune tolerance lasts 1 to 3 decades and patients respond poorly to treatment with interferon.

- Immune clearance: This is the first phase of chronic hepatitis B acquired in late childhood and adulthood and the second phase in perinatally acquired infection. It is characterized by the presence of HBe Ag seroconversion. This seroconversion may be accompanied by an increase in ALT due to immune-mediated hepatocyte destruction and an increase in the HBV DNA. These exacerbations, which can be severe in some cases, are associated with an increase in the anti-HBc IgM antibody and may be misdiagnosed as acute hepatitis. In some cases, patients may not clear the HBe Ag completely and may have intermittent disappearance of HBV DNA and HBe Ag. These patients are at increased risk of cirrhosis and hepatocellular carcinoma.

- Nonreplicative phase: These patients are HBs Ag positive and HBe Ag negative with antibody to HBe Ag. These patients, in whom there is no viral replication, no HBV DNA in the serum, no inflammation on liver biopsy, and normal ALT, are referred to as inactive carriers. These patients may clear HBs Ag but remain at risk for cirrhosis and hepatocellular carcinoma because even though there is no detectable HBV DNA in the serum it is detectable with polymerase chain reaction (PCR). This may be due to persistent low level of viral replication or infection with wild-type hepatitis B virus or hepatitis B variants resulting in decreased HBs Ag production. When these patients are immunosuppressed, reactivation of hepatitis B with reappearance of HBe Ag and HBV DNA can occur.

Clinical Manifestations

- Patients may be completely asymptomatic or have nonspecific symptoms such as fatigue.
- Flares of chronic hepatitis B present with right upper quadrant discomfort and jaundice similar to acute hepatitis.
- Some patients have extrahepatic manifestations similar to serum sickness seen with acute hepatitis B with fever, arthralgia, and skin rash.
- Chronic hepatitis B is associated with polyarteritis nodosa and membranous glomerulonephritis.

Diagnosis

Serology: Presented in Table 6-2.

Treatment

- The aim of treatment is the sustained suppression of HBV replication (seroconversion of HBe Ag) and remission of liver disease. Response is characterized as virologic (decrease in HBV DNA to less than 100,000 copies/mL or 2 log reduction from

TABLE 6-2 Serology of Acute Hepatitis B

	HBs Ag	Anti HBs	Anti-HBc Antibody	HBe Ag	Anti-HBe Antibody	HBV DNA
Acute hepatitis B (early)	+	−	−	+	−	+
Acute hepatitis B (window period)	+	−	IgM	+	−	+/−
Acute hepatitis B (recovery)	+	+	IgG	−	+	−
Chronic hepatitis B, high replication	+	−	IgG	+	−	+
Chronic hepatitis B, low/nonreplicative phase	+	−	IgG	−	+	−
Chronic hepatitis B precore mutant	+	−	IgG	−	+	+
Chronic hepatitis B inactive carrier	+	−	IgG	−	+/−	Low-level +
Chronic hepatitis B reactivation	+	−	IgM	+	−	+
Hepatitis B vaccine	−	+	−	−	−	−

From Yamada T, Alpers D, Kaplowitz N, et al. *Textbook of gastroenterology*. 4th ed. Baltimore: Lippincott Williams & Wilkins; 2003:942, with permission.

baseline), biochemical (decrease in ALT to normal), or histologic (improved histology on two consecutive liver biopsies).

- Patients with chronic hepatitis B who are HBe Ag positive and have high HBV DNA > 10^5 copies/mL and normal ALT can be followed with serial ALT every 3 months. If the ALT is greater than twice the upper limit of normal or persistently elevated ALT after 6 months, patients should have a liver biopsy and initiate treatment.
- Inactive chronic hepatitis B carriers (HBs Ag positive, HBe Ag negative, and normal ALT) can be followed with ALT every 6 months, if ALT > 2 times normal, HBV DNA levels should be checked
- Three approved treatments for hepatitis B are interferon, lamivudine, and adefovir.
- Interferon alpha has antiviral, antiproliferative, and immunomodulatory effects. Side effects include leukopenia, flulike effects, fever, depression, and skin rash.
- Lamivudine is an orally administered nucleoside analogue that inhibits HBV replication. Randomized double-blind

placebo-controlled trials have shown that 1 year treatment with lamivudine resulted in HBe Ag seroconversion in 18% of patients compared to 6% in controls. Lamivudine has been shown to prevent cirrhosis in patients with chronic hepatitis B, reverse fibrosis seen in patients with cirrhosis, and reverse decompensated cirrhosis. The limitation of lamivudine is the development of resistance due to mutations with up to 25% at 1 year and close to 70% resistance with 4 years of therapy. Side effects include headache, fatigue, nausea, pancreatitis, and peripheral neuropathy.
- Adefovir is a reverse transcriptase inhibitor that inhibits DNA polymerase. Resistance with adefovir has also been noted but is lower than with lamivudine. Adefovir resistance has been 0% at 1 year, 2% to 5% at 2 years, and 18% at 4 years. Patients should be monitored for nephrotoxicity.
- Entecavir and telbivudine are new oral nucleoside analogues that have been approved for treatment of chronic hepatitis B.

Recommendations for Hepatocellular Carcinoma Screening

- High-risk hepatitis B carriers, i.e., those older than 45 years, patients with family history of hepatocellular carcinoma (HCC), and patients with cirrhosis should have serial follow up with alternating 6 months alpha-fetoprotein (AFP) and USG.
- Low-risk patients should be considered for screening especially those from endemic areas.

Prognosis

Cirrhosis develops in 0.1% to 2% of patients with chronic hepatitis B per year. In patients with cirrhosis the risk for progression to HCC is between 2% and 10% per year.

Acute Hepatitis C

Epidemiology/Pathogenesis

- Hepatitis C virus (HVC) is a single-stranded RNA virus of the Flavivirus family.
- HCV accounts for one fifth of all cases of acute hepatitis.
- HCV virus is spread by the blood and therefore the majority of cases are caused by intravenous drug use and blood transfusions. HCV can be transmitted sexually but transmission has been found to be rare. Perinatal transmission of HCV is related to the presence of viremia at the time of birth. There is no evidence to support the transmission of HCV by breastfeeding.
- Incubation period of hepatitis C ranges from 4 to 24 weeks.

Clinical Manifestations

- Most patients are asymptomatic.
- Clinical manifestations are similar to all other forms of hepatitis with fatigue, malaise, nausea, vomiting, jaundice, right upper quadrant pain, dark urine, and clay-colored stool. Symptoms last 2 to 12 weeks.
- In rare cases adults present with fulminant hepatic failure and encephalopathy.

Physical Examination

- Icterus
- Tender hepatomegaly

Diagnosis

- Liver function tests
  - Elevated transaminases (ALT > AST ~ 1000 IU/L) 6 to 12 weeks following exposure
- Serology (Fig. 6-6)
  - HCV RNA is detectable within 1 to 2 weeks following exposure.
  - Antibody to HCV is not protective and becomes positive 8 to 10 weeks following exposure.

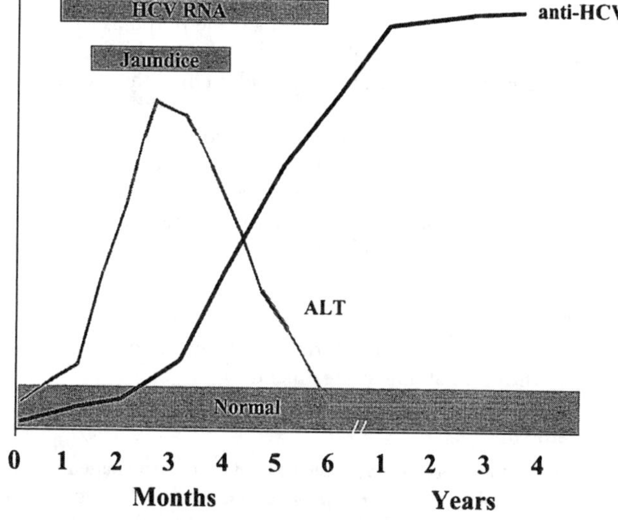

Figure 6-6 • Typical serologic course of acute hepatitis C virus infection. (From Yamada T, Alpers D, Kaplowitz N, et al. *Textbook of gastroenterology*. Vol. 2. 4th ed. Baltimore: Lippincott Williams & Wilkins; 2003:2291, with permission.)

Treatment/Prognosis

- Patients who do not spontaneously clear HCV by 12 weeks are unlikely to clear HCV.
- 80% of patients with acute hepatitis C develop chronic hepatitis and 20% of patients with chronic hepatitis develop cirrhosis after 10 years.
- There is limited evidence to support the use of interferon-alpha in patients with acute hepatitis C.

Chronic Hepatitis C

Of patients with acute hepatitis C, 80% develop chronic hepatitis C.

Clinical Manifestations

- Most patients are asymptomatic or have nonspecific symptoms like fatigue and myalgia.
- Patients may have abdominal pain and jaundice.
- Extrahepatic manifestations are less common than in patients with hepatitis B.
- These extrahepatic manifestations include the following:
  - Essential mixed cryoglobulinemia: Deposition of immune complexes in small to medium-sized blood vessels resulting in a small vessel vasculitis with palpable purpura, weakness and arthralgia, peripheral neuropathy, and renal failure.
  - Autoimmune disorders: Hypothyroidism from the production of antithyroid peroxidase antibodies.
  - Skin disease: Porphyria cutanea tarda, leukocytoclastic vasculitis, lichen planus, and necrolytic acral erythema.
  - Renal disease: Glomerulonephritis secondary to mixed cryoglobulinemia, membranoproliferative glomerulonephritis, or membranous glomerulonephritis.

Diagnosis

Liver biopsy is of utility in determining the extent of fibrosis and thereby the optimal time of treatment.

Treatment

- Treatment for hepatitis C should be considered in all patients with increased risk of progression (patients with HCV DNA, fibrosis on liver biopsy, or elevated ALT). In patients with mild disease (grade A) treatment can be deferred, whereas if biopsy results show moderate to severe disease treatment should be initiated. Treatment for hepatitis C consists of interferon and ribavirin.

- Sustained viral response (SVR) is defined as the presence of undetectable HCV RNA 6 months off treatment. Response to therapy varies with hepatitis C genotype. Patients with genotype I are more refractory to therapy than patients with genotype II or III.
- Early virologic response (EVR), defined as a 2 log reduction in HCV RNA levels or no detectable serum HCV RNA in 3 months, has been shown to be predictive of response to treatment.
- Phase III trails are currently under way using valopicitabine (NM 283) a prodrug of a novel ribonucleoside analogue in patients with refractory hepatitis C.
- Patients with chronic hepatitis C should be advised to avoid alcohol and medications should be dosed for liver disease.
- Vaccination for hepatitis A and B, pneumococcus, and annual influenza is indicated.

Prognosis

- Cirrhosis develops in 50% of patients with chronic hepatitis C or at the rate of 0.1% to 7% per year.
- HCC occurs at the rate of 1% to 4% per year and occurs exclusively in patients with hepatitis C who have developed cirrhosis.

Screening

- Patients with cirrhosis should be screened for esophageal varices.
- HCC screening with 6-month alternating AFP and abdominal USG.

Hepatitis D Infection

- Hepatitis D virus (HDV) or hepatitis delta virus is an incomplete RNA virus that requires hepatitis B virus for replication. The HD virion consists of the hepatitis delta antigen surrounded by an envelope of hepatitis B. Hepatitis D is transmitted by the same route as hepatitis B: through blood products, injection drug use, and sexual transmission. Perinatal transmission, however, is rare in hepatitis D.
- Acute infection with hepatitis D can occur with hepatitis B coinfection or superinfection in chronic hepatitis B carriers. The clinical presentation is indistinguishable from other causes of acute hepatitis; however, serology can help differentiate hepatitis D from other viruses and coinfection from superinfection.

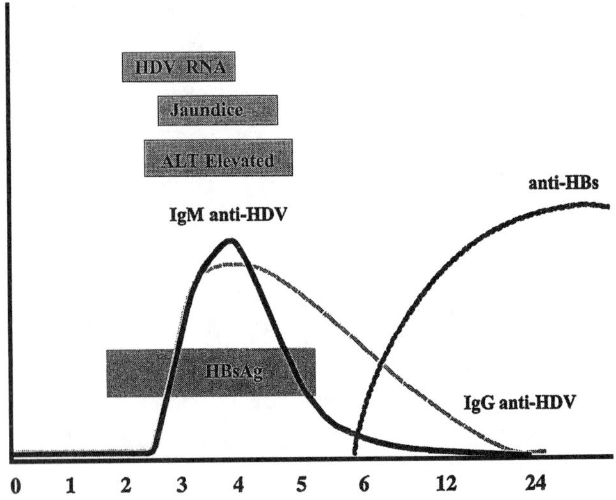

Figure 6-7 • Typical serologic course of acute hepatitis D virus coinfection. (From Yamada T, Alpers D, Kaplowitz N, et al. *Textbook of gastroenterology*. Vol. 2. 4th ed. Baltimore: Lippincott Williams & Wilkins; 2003:2291, with permission.)

- In coinfection of hepatitis D and hepatitis B, markers of hepatitis B are detected earlier than markers of hepatitis D. HBsAg and anti-HBc antibody are detected early in the disease, hepatitis D antigen in 1 to 2 weeks followed by IgM antihepatitis D antibody (Fig. 6-7).
- In hepatitis D superinfection, hepatitis D antigen and IgM and IgG to hepatitis D are detected early during the symptomatic phase in addition to HBs antigen. In contrast to coinfection, anti-HBc antibody is not detected (Fig. 6-8).

Hepatitis E

Hepatitis E virus (HEV) is a nonenveloped RNA virus transmitted by fecal–oral route. Cases are rare in the United States and are mainly seen in individuals who travel to endemic areas. Hepatitis E has been responsible for outbreaks of hepatitis that have been self-limited except in pregnant women who can develop fulminant hepatic failure. Diagnosis of hepatitis E is with the detection of anti-HEV IgM, which is detectable early in the symptomatic phase and remains positive for 1 to 2 months. Anti-HEV IgG is detectable after recovery and may be protective for a limited duration. Treatment of hepatitis E is supportive; prevention of hepatitis E outbreaks is with purification of drinking water.

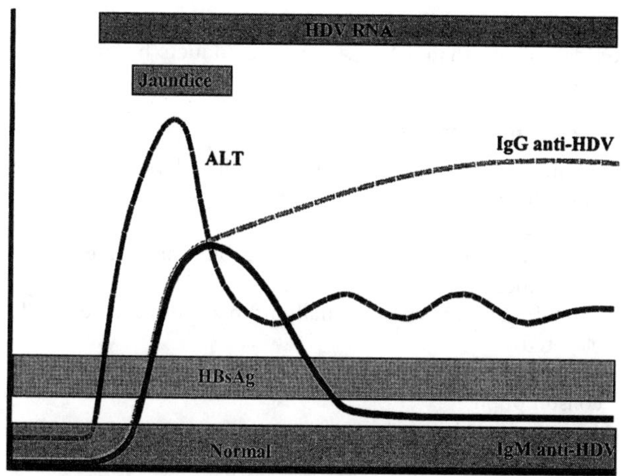

Figure 6-8 • Typical serologic course of acute hepatitis D virus superinfection. (From Yamada T, Alpers D, Kaplowitz N, et al. *Textbook of gastroenterology*. Vol. 2. 4th ed. Baltimore: Lippincott Williams & Wilkins; 2003:2291, with permission.)

Differential Diagnosis

Wilson's disease, CMV, EBV infection, autoimmune hepatitis, drug toxicity, and in pregnant women acute fatty liver of pregnancy and HELLP (hemolysis, elevated liver enzymes and low platelets) should be considered.

ALCOHOLIC LIVER DISEASE

Daily intake of ethanol of 40 g in men or 20 g in women over greater than 10 years results in a significant increase in the incidence of cirrhosis. The peak incidence of alcoholic liver disease (ALD) is in the third decade in women and in the fourth decade in men. Women develop alcohol-induced liver disease with smaller doses of alcohol and have a more rapid progression of liver disease than men.

Mechanisms of Injury Secondary to Alcohol

- Ethanol metabolism consumes oxygen depriving hepatocytes around the central vein of oxygen and thereby resulting in hepatocyte necrosis.
- Polymorphonuclear cell infiltration with release of free radicals.
- Elevated lipopolysaccharide absorption from the gut and activation of Kupffer cells by the oxidation of ethanol.

- Acetaldehyde and hydroxyethyl radicals derived from the oxidation of ethanol form antigenic adducts by binding to proteins.

Clinical Manifestations

The clinical presentation secondary to ethanol use ranges from fatty liver to cirrhosis.

- Alcoholic fatty liver
  - Patients are usually asymptomatic but may have tender hepatomegaly.
  - Liver function tests are usually normal but may be mildly elevated.
  - Fatty liver is usually reversible with cessation of alcohol consumption.
- Alcoholic hepatitis
  - Patients present with anorexia, weakness, weight loss, fever, and jaundice.
  - Abdominal pain is rare.
  - Physical exam is notable for tender hepatomegaly, icterus. Patients may have signs of chronic liver disease with palmar erythema, spider nevi, gynecomastia, testicular atrophy, and parotid enlargement.
  - Laboratory data are notable for AST > ALT (2:1), elevated bilirubin, alkaline phosphatase (usually not greater than 300 IU/L), elevated γ-glutamyl transferase (GGT) and low albumin. Alcoholic hepatitis has been shown to progress to cirrhosis even with cessation of alcohol consumption.
- Cirrhosis
  - Patients may also present with complications of liver disease including spontaneous bacterial peritonitis, hepatorenal syndrome, and variceal bleeding.
  - Physical exam is notable for signs of chronic liver disease and portal hypertension with splenomegaly, caput medusae, and ascites.
  - Laboratory data are notable for increased transaminases with AST > ALT (2:1), elevated bilirubin, alkaline phosphatase, and GGT. GGT is elevated due to the induction by alcohol. Poor synthetic function results in low albumin and elevated prothrombin time.

Diagnosis

- History: It is important to obtain a detailed and accurate history of the extent of alcohol use, risk factors for hepatitis, and medications that may be hepatotoxic.
- Rule out concurrent causes of liver disease such as hepatitis, hemochromatosis and autoimmune hepatitis.

- Liver biopsy: This is indicated in patients in whom the diagnosis is uncertain, patients with concurrent liver disease from another etiology, and to determine the prognosis of ALD.

Prognosis

- Alcoholic fatty liver carries a good prognosis with reversal of disease with abstinence.
- Risk scores have been developed to estimate the prognosis in patients with ALD. Two such scores are:
  Discriminant function = (4.6 × [prothrombin time—control PT]) + (serum bilirubin). A discriminant function >32 is associated with a high mortality and should be treated with corticosteroids.
- Mortality in end-stage liver disease (MELD) score is based on bilirubin, isoniazid (INR), and creatinine. The MELD score is a formula to predict short-term mortality in patients with end-stage chronic liver disease and is used to prioritize patients for liver transplantation. The score has been shown to be as useful as the discriminant function in predicting mortality in patients with alcoholic hepatitis.

Treatment

- Abstinence from alcohol.
- Vaccination with hepatitis A, B, and pneumococcal vaccine, and annual influenza vaccine is indicated.
- Corticosteroids in severe alcoholic hepatitis if discriminant score >35 or encephalopathy. Prednisolone is preferred to prednisone, which needs to be converted to prednisolone by the liver.
- Liver transplant in patients with chronic liver disease who have been abstinent for 6 months.
- Nutritional support: Short-term enteral feeding in patients with decompensated liver disease decreases mortality and Child–Pugh score. Long-term nutritional supplementation has been shown to decrease frequency of hospitalizations and infections.

CIRRHOSIS

Cirrhosis of the liver is characterized by necrosis, fibrosis, and hepatic regeneration with resultant loss of architecture.

Etiology/Pathogenesis

Cirrhosis has been classified according to morphology, etiology, and histology separately but each classification has limitations. The most clinically useful classification of cirrhosis is as follows:

- Alcoholic cirrhosis
- Biliary cirrhosis
- Cardiac cirrhosis
- Metabolic and toxic
- Cryptogenic and posthepatic

Clinical Manifestations

- Patients may be completely asymptomatic or have nonspecific symptoms with anorexia, nausea, malnutrition, and weight loss.
- Patients may have symptoms secondary to complications of hepatocellular dysfunction with jaundice, altered mental status secondary to hepatic encephalopathy, bleeding secondary to coagulopathy, and edema from hypoalbuminemia.
- Patients may present with complications from portal hypertension with variceal bleeding, ascites, or spontaneous bacterial peritonitis.

Physical Examination

- Nodular liver that may be enlarged, normal, or shrunken.
- Scleral icterus is visible when the bilirubin is greater than 2 mg/dL.
- Parotid and lacrimal gland enlargement.
- *Fetor hepaticus*: Pungent odor to the breath due to increased concentrations of dimethyl sulfide.
- Skin: Spider angiomata on the upper extremities, face, and chest.
- Hand/nail: Palmar erythema, Dupuytren contractures from thickening of the palmar fascia, clubbing. Muehrcke nails are transverse white bands across the nails. They represent an abnormality in the vascular bed and disappear when pressure is applied to the nail. Terry's nails are characterized by a white appearance of the proximal two-thirds while the distal one-third is red. Terry's nails are not specific to cirrhosis and can be seen in hypoalbuminemia.
- Ascites
- Splenomegaly
- *Caput medusae*: Secondary to portal hypertension there is increased flow in the obliterated periumbilical, umbilical, and anterior abdominal wall veins.
- Asterixis: Not specific to patients with hepatic failure and may be seen with uremia and heart failure.

Laboratory Findings

- Elevated transaminases: AST > ALT; however, they can be normal. In early stages of chronic liver disease ALT > AST and reversal of transaminases AST > ALT occurs with cirrhosis.

- Elevated alkaline phosphatase and GGT (two to three times the upper limit of normal).
- Elevated bilirubin in decompensated cirrhosis.
- Albumin is decreased and prothrombin time elevated due to poor synthetic function of the liver.
- Anemia secondary to iron or folate deficiency, blood loss, anemia of chronic disease, and direct toxic effects of alcohol on the bone marrow.
- Thrombocytopenia secondary splenomegaly in patients with portal hypertension and splenic sequestration.

Diagnosis

- History of alcohol, drug use, risk factors for hepatitis, family history of neuropsychiatric diseases, skin hyperpigmentation, diabetes, cardiomyopathy, and liver disease should all be sought.
- Serology for hepatitis B, hepatitis C; iron studies to rule out hemochromatosis (iron, total iron-binding capacity, ferritin); serum copper and ceruloplasmin to rule out Wilson's disease; antimitochondrial antibody to rule out primary biliary cirrhosis; antismooth muscle, antiliver kidney microsomal, antinuclear antibody for autoimmune hepatitis and primary sclerosing cholangitis, and serum alpha-1-antitrypsin.
- Liver biopsy: The most sensitive test in diagnosing cirrhosis and is of value in determining the etiology of cirrhosis.

Complications

Ascites

Ascites is one of the first manifestations of alcoholic liver disease and may fluctuate corresponding to periods of alcohol ingestion. In nonalcoholic cirrhosis, ascites develops at a late stage.

- Evaluation of ascitic fluid by paracentesis is useful in determining the etiology of the ascites and in ruling out infection.
- Components of ascitic fluid and interpretation:
  - Ascitic fluid should be analyzed for cell count with differential, albumin, total protein, gram stain, and culture in all cases. In special cases, glucose, lactate dehydrogenase (LDH), amylase, cytology, and acid-fast stain for tuberculosis (TB) should be considered.
  - Cell count: Upper limit of normal white cell count <500 cells/mm^3 with a polymorphonuclear (PMN) count of <250 cells/mm^3. Total cell counts can increase with diuresis but the absolute PMN count should be <250 cell/mm^3. The PMN count should be corrected for traumatic taps with 1 PMN for every 250 red blood cells and 1 lymphocyte per 750 red cells. TB peritonitis should be suspected if the ascitic fluid is mononuclear cell predominant.

- Serum ascitis albumin gradient (SAAG) = Serum albumin–Ascites albumin. The SAAG is a measure of portal pressure with a gradient of >1.1 g/dL suggestive of portal hypertension, and conversely SAAG < 1.1 is suggestive of a cause of ascites related to nonportal hypertension. SAAG can be artificially low in the case of severe hypoalbuminemia (serum albumin < 1.1 g/dL) and in patients with hypotension as portal pressure is low. SAAG may be artificially high in patients with chylous ascites.

- Total protein: Determination of the total protein is of value in two cases:
  - Patients with cirrhosis and ascitic protein <1 g/dL are more likely to have spontaneous bacterial peritonitis (SBP) and should be on prophylaxis with a fluoroquinolone.
  - To distinguish SBP from gut perforation into ascitic fluid.
- Ascitic fluid with two of three of the following is suggestive of a perforation: ascitic fluid glucose < 50 mg/dL, an LDH > upper limit of normal, and total protein >1 g/dL. Gram stain of ascitic fluid is of utility when positive and in cases where bowel perforation is suspected.
- Acid-fast bacilli (AFB) stain for TB and culture: Limited sensitivity (2% and 40%, respectively) and peritoneal biopsy (up to 80% sensitive) may be indicated in patients with high index of suspicion.
- Amylase: Ascitic fluid amylase concentration is 40 IU/L ± 40 IU/L in uncomplicated cirrhotic ascites, and the ascitic fluid/serum amylase is approximately 0.4. Pancreatic ascites and bowel perforation are associated with higher amylase concentrations.
- Special tests based on ascitic fluid appearance: Ascitic fluid that is milky in appearance should be tested for triglycerides. Chylous ascites should be suspected if triglyceride concentration is >200 mg/dL. Brown ascitic fluid should be tested for bilirubin. Levels that are higher that serum bilirubin suggest a bowel or biliary perforation.

Infection of Ascitic Fluid

This should be suspected in patients with fever, abdominal pain/tenderness, altered mental status. Infection of ascitic fluid can be classified on the basis of the number of polymorphonuclear cells and cultures as:

	PMN/ mm^3	Culture
Spontaneous bacterial peritonitis	>250	One microorganism
Culture-negative neutrocytic ascites (CNNA)	>250	No growth
Secondary bacterial peritonitis	>250	Multiple organisms
Monomicrobial bacterascites	<250	Single organism
Polymicrobial bacterascites	<250	Multiple organisms

Spontaneous Bacterial Peritonitis (>250 Cells/mm^3 and One Microorganism)

Etiology/Pathogenesis

- Spontaneous infection of ascitic fluid in SBP occurs secondary to translocation of gut flora. Bacteria enter the local lymph nodes and subsequently the vasculature. The resultant lymph that forms ascites contains these bacteria, which fail to be opsonized in the protein-deficient ascitic fluid resulting in SBP.
- The most common organisms are *Escherichia coli*, *Streptococcus pneumoniae*, and *Klebsiella pneumoniae*.
- Patients with cirrhosis from alcohol use and hepatitis develop SBP. However, SBP is rare in patients with cardiac cirrhosis and patients with malignant ascites.

Clinical Manifestations

- Predisposing factors include bacteremia from any source including urinary tract infections, gastrointestinal bleeding due to transmigration of bowel flora in areas of injured mucosa, or from resultant endoscopic procedure.
- SBP should be suspected in patients with cirrhosis who develop fever, abdominal pain, altered mental status, diarrhea, ileus, hypotension, or leukocytosis.

Diagnosis

- Paracentesis is the diagnostic procedure of choice and should be performed if there is any suspicion of SBP.
- As mentioned in the table above, patients with PMN > 250/mm^3 and one organism on culture have SBP. An adjusted PMN count should be calculated in patients with bloody ascites with 1 PMN subtracted for every 250 red cells. If the calculated PMN > 250/mm^3, then SBP should be considered.

Treatment

- Third-generation cephalosporin such as cefotaxime. Duration of treatment is determined by the clinical response. If abdominal pain and fever resolve, the antibiotics can be discontinued in 5 days. However, if symptoms persist, repeat paracentesis is necessary. If the repeat cell count is less than 250 cells/mm^3, then treatment is discontinued. If it is higher than 250 and more than the pretreatment value, antibiotics are continued and repeat paracenteses are used to guide duration of therapy.
- Prevention of renal failure: Acute renal failure develops in one third of patients with SBP. It is hypothesized that renal failure results from the activation of the renin–angiotensin system with decreased renal perfusion and may be mitigated by treatment

with intravenous infusions of albumin (1.5 mg/kg of bodyweight at the time of diagnosis followed by 1 mg/kg after day 3)

Prevention

- Prophylaxis for SBP is indicated in patients with prior episodes of SBP because recurrence rates are high.
- In patients with acute variceal bleeding, treatment with oral norfloxacin (400 mg BID for 7 days) or intravenous ciprofloxacin with oral amoxicillin + clavulanic acid for 7 days has been shown to prevent SBP and improve survival (Rimola et al. *J Hepatol.* 2003;32:142–153).
- In patients with ascitic fluid protein concentration <15 g/dL, indefinite treatment with norfloxacin or ciprofloxacin has been shown to decrease the risk of a first episode of SBP. However, it has not been shown to improve survival.

Secondary Bacterial Peritonitis (>250 Cells/mm^3 and Multiple Organisms on Culture)

- Diagnosis is suggested by two of three of the following in the ascitic fluid analysis: total protein >1 g/dL, glucose < 50 mg/dL, LDH > 225 mU/mL.
- Emergent computed tomography (CT) should be performed in patients with secondary bacterial peritonitis to localize the source of perforation.
- Treatment consists of antibiotics and surgery.

Culture-Negative Neutrocytic Ascites (>250 Cells/mm^3 and No Growth)

- Following initial paracentesis given the elevated PMN count in ascitic fluid, patients are started on antibiotics. However, by definition in patients with CNNA ascitic fluid cultures show no growth.
- To guide treatment, repeat paracentesis should be performed. If cell count has decreased, then antibiotics should be continued for 5 days. No change in PMN count despite antibiotics suggests a nonbacterial cause of CNNA, and biopsy and cultures for AFB should be considered.

Monomicrobial Bacterascites (<250 Cells/mm^3 and No Growth)

- Patients who have convincing signs or symptoms of an infection should be treated empirically irrespective of the PMN count. If cultures remain negative for 48 h, antibiotics can be discontinued.

- In patients with monomicrobial nonneutrocytic bacterascites without symptoms, paracentesis can be repeated, and if the PMN count is elevated >250, should be treated.

Hepatopulmonary Syndrome

Patients with hepatopulmonary syndrome (HPS) present with the classic triad of liver disease, intrapulmonary vascular dilatation, and an elevated alveolar–arterial gradient while breathing room air.

Pathogenesis

- Hypoxia in HPS is secondary to intrapulmonary shunting of blood, alveolar ventilation/pulmonary perfusion (V/Q) mismatch and decreased oxygen diffusion secondary to intrapulmonary vascular dilatation, and loss of hypoxic vasoconstriction. These vascular abnormalities are a consequence of inhibition of vasoconstrictors and decreased clearance of vasodilators by the liver. The severity of hypoxia is unrelated to the degree of liver disease.
- Unlike the case with true shunts, patients with HPS intrapulmonary shunts improve partially with increasing inspired oxygen concentration.

Clinical Manifestations

- Patients have dyspnea at rest.
- Platynea is defined as increased dyspnea with sitting up and improvement in recumbent position.
- Increase in dyspnea with sitting up is due to the redistribution of blood in the lower lobes.
- Orthodeoxia is defined as arterial desaturation with sitting up and improvement in recumbent position.

Diagnosis

- A-a (alveolar arterial) gradient > 15 to 20 mm Hg measured with the patient in sitting position.
- Chest radiograph: Usually normal but may show increased vascular markings in the lower lobes.
- Pulmonary function testing: In the absence of coexisting lung disease, patients may have normal lung volumes or have restrictive lung disease secondary to ascites. Diffusion capacity for carbon monoxide (DLCO) is decreased.
- Bubble or contrast echocardiography: Microbubbles produced by agitated saline or contrast injected peripherally result in opacification of the right heart and are filtered by the pulmonary capillaries. However, in the presence of an intracardiac or intrapulmonary shunt, contrast appears in the left heart. In an intracardiac right to left shunt, dye or bubbles appear within

three heartbeats in the left heart, whereas in an intrapulmonary shunt they are seen in the left chambers in three to six heartbeats.
- Macroaggregated albumin scan: Albumin macroaggregates are normally filtered in the pulmonary vascular bed, and their presence in the brain or kidneys suggests the presence of a shunt.
- Pulmonary angiography: Rarely necessary; performed only to exclude other causes of hypoxia.

Treatment

- Supplemental oxygen.
- Liver transplant is the only proven treatment for hepatopulmonary syndrome.

Hepatorenal Syndrome

Hepatorenal syndrome is defined as the development of acute renal failure in patients with advanced liver disease secondary to severe vasoconstriction of renal circulation.

Pathophysiology

- Hepatorenal syndrome results from decreased renal perfusion from underfilling of arterial circulation.
- Decreased renal perfusion results in activation of the renin–angiotensin system with consequent renal vasoconstriction and further decrease in perfusion. This renal hypoperfusion secondary to vasoconstriction occurs in the setting of systemic and splanchnic vasodilatation mediated by the endothelium-derived relaxation factor, nitric oxide.

Diagnostic Criteria Proposed by the International Ascites Club

- Advanced chronic or acute liver failure with portal hypertension
- Serum creatinine greater than 1.5 mg/dL or creatinine clearance lower than 40 mL/min
- The absence of shock, bacterial infection, nephrotoxic drug exposure, or rapid loss of fluid through the gut or kidneys
- No sustained improvement in renal function with withdrawal of diuretics and plasma expansion with 1.5 L of isotonic saline
- Proteinuria less than 500 mg/day and no ultrasound evidence of obstructive uropathy or parenchymal renal disease

Clinical Manifestations

- Spontaneous bacterial peritonitis may precipitate hepatorenal syndrome
- Patients initially have normal urine output
- Oliguria and anuria represent a preterminal event
- Hepatorenal syndrome has been classified based on the clinical presentation as follows:

- Type I: 50% decrease in creatinine clearance to <20 mL/min in less than 2 weeks or twofold increase in serum creatinine to a level >2.5 mg/dL
- Type II: Less severe renal insufficiency that does not meet criteria for type I hepatorenal syndrome

Diagnosis (Fig. 6-9)

- Urine analysis
- Renal ultrasound

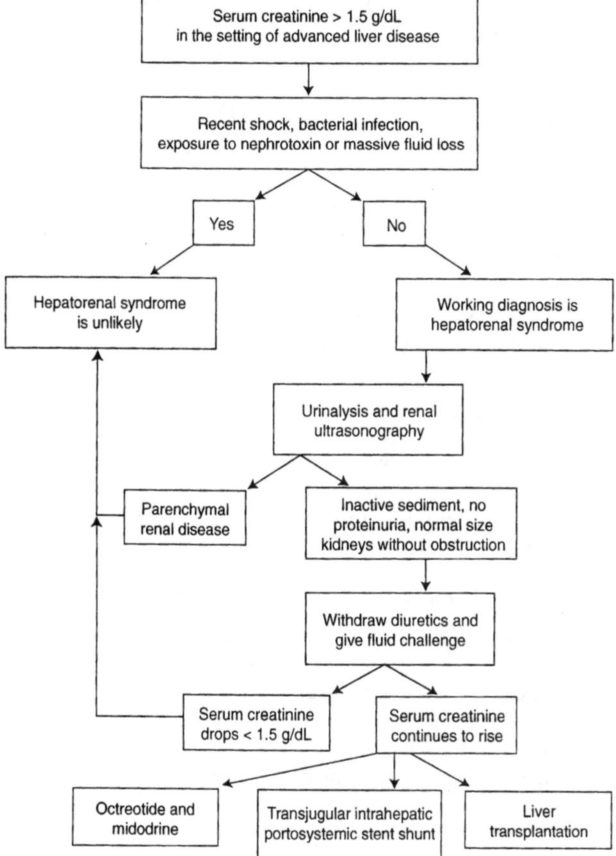

Figure 6-9 • Algorithm for the diagnosis and treatment of patients with suspected hepatorenal syndrome. (From Yamada T, Alpers D, Kaplowitz N, et al. *Textbook of gastroenterology*. Vol. 1. 4th ed. Baltimore: Lippincott Williams & Wilkins; 2003:968, with permission.)

Treatment

- Vasoactive agents: Clonidine in the acute stage decreases sympathetic tone and renal vascular resistance. Limited data with combined therapy with octreotide and midodrine (alpha-1 agonist) may be effective in improving renal function.
- Transjugular intrahepatic portasystemic shunt (TIPS) is effective in relieving portal hypertension and in case series has been shown to decrease creatinine. However, TIPS should be reserved for patients with MELD score <18.
- Hemodialysis should be considered in patients awaiting liver transplantation and continuous venovenous filtration in patients in whom blood pressure may be a limiting factor.
- Liver transplantation.

Prevention

- Intravenous albumin: Patients with SBP benefit from treatment with intravenous albumin. A dose of 1.5 g/kg of albumin at the time of diagnosis of SBP and another dose of 1.0 g/kg on day 3 of treatment may reduce renal impairment that does not reverse during hospitalization and decrease mortality both during hospitalization and at 3 months (Sort et al. *N Engl J Med.* 1999;341:403–409).
- Pentoxyphylline: May decrease the incidence of hepatorenal syndrome in patients with alcoholic hepatitis.

Wilson's Disease

An autosomal recessive disorder characterized by a defect in copper transport localized to chromosome 13. This defect involves a copper-transporting protein in the liver thereby resulting in the accumulation of copper in the liver and other organs.

Etiology/Pathogenesis

- Copper is bound to apoceruloplasmin in the liver forming ceruloplasmin and circulates in the plasma.
- Copper is excreted into the bile and excreted in the stool. Only a small proportion is excreted by the kidneys.
- Patients with Wilson's disease have defective excretion of copper by the liver into the biliary tree.

Clinical Manifestations

- Patients are asymptomatic until 5 years of age after which asymptomatic elevation in liver function tests may be seen.
- Neuropsychiatric manifestations: Ataxia, tremor, rigidity, slurred speech, depression, and schizophrenia.

- Ocular manifestations: Accumulation of copper in the cornea results in the characteristic green-brown pigmentation in the periphery called Kayser–Fleischer ring that can be seen on slit lamp examination. Sunflower cataracts due to deposition of copper in the lens may be seen.
- Hepatic manifestations: Include asymptomatic elevation in liver function tests, acute hepatitis, chronic active hepatitis, fulminant hepatic failure, and cirrhosis.
- Acute hepatitis is indistinguishable from other causes of hepatitis, often resolves spontaneously, and can therefore be missed.
- Fulminant hepatic failure with rapid onset of jaundice, liver failure with coagulopathy and encephalopathy.
- The presence of Coombs negative hemolytic anemia due to the release of copper from the liver in fulminant hepatic failure is characteristic of Wilson's disease.

Diagnosis

- Elevated serum aminotransferases with ALT > AST. Patients with fulminant hepatic failure from Wilson's disease may have inappropriately mild elevation of transaminases and low serum alkaline phosphatase with elevated bilirubin.
- Low serum ceruloplasmin is not sensitive or specific for Wilson's disease.
- Elevated serum copper levels are not sensitive for diagnosing Wilson's disease but can be used for monitoring response to therapy.
- Urine copper: High variability in urine copper makes spot urine copper levels an unreliable test; 24-h urine collection >100 μg is seen in Wilson's disease and other liver diseases. Urinary copper measurement after a penicillamine challenge is a more specific test for diagnosing Wilson's disease.
- Elevated hepatic copper content (>250 μg/g dry weight) is the gold standard.

Treatment

- Removal of copper from the liver: Copper chelating agents such as penicillamine or trientine.
- Maintenance therapy to prevent reaccumulation of copper: Low-dose copper chelators or oral zinc that prevents copper absorption.
- Patients with fulminant hepatic failure must be referred for urgent liver transplant. While awaiting transplant hemodialysis, plasmapheresis or exchange transfusion is needed.
- First-degree relatives of patients with Wilson's disease should have screening physical and laboratory evaluation of liver function.

Hemochromatosis

Hereditary hemochromatosis (HH) is an autosomal recessive disorder characterized by increased absorption of intestinal iron resulting in iron overload. C282Y and H63D are the most common mutations in the *HFE* gene.

Etiology/Pathogenesis

- 10% of 10 to 20 mg of dietary iron is absorbed from the gut to match GI and skin losses of 1 mg/day.
- In normal subjects, absorption of both heme and nonheme iron is regulated by iron stores in the form of ferritin.
- In hemochromatosis there is no negative feedback leading to progressive accumulation in the liver and other organs.

Clinical Manifestations

- Onset of symptoms is in the fourth to fifth decade in men. Women present later due to the iron losses from menstruation and increased requirement in pregnancy and lactation.
- Liver: Hepatomegaly, cirrhosis, and increased risk of hepatocellular carcinoma (20-fold increased risk).
- Pancreas: Diabetes mellitus
- Skin: Characteristic hyperpigmentation of the skin
- Joints: Pseudogout with deposition of calcium pyrophosphate crystals and classic chondrocalcinosis. Metacarpophalangeal joints narrowing and hooklike osteophytes on the radial aspect are characteristic of pseudogout in HH.
- Heart: Dilated cardiomyopathy and conduction system abnormalities due to the deposition of iron in the myocardium.
- Pituitary: Hypogonadism due to decreased production of trophic hormones and less commonly from deposition in the testicles. Decreased testosterone in men results in diminished libido and impotence.
- Increased susceptibility to infections: Increased iron in macrophages results in decreased phagocytosis and patients are susceptible to *Yersinia enterocolitica*, *Vibrio vulnificus*, and *Listeria* infections.

Diagnosis

- Iron studies: Fasting iron studies that include plasma iron, total iron binding capacity (transferrin), and ferritin. Fasting transferrin saturation (iron/transferrin) $\geq$ 60% in men and 50% in women is suggestive of iron overload secondary to hemochromatosis, and genetic testing should be pursued.
- *Genetic testing:* Evaluation for *HFE* mutations C282Y and H63D.

- *Liver biopsy*: Indicated in patients with elevated liver function tests, ferritin > 1000 mg/dL or compound heterozygotes with C282Y/H63D since they have a higher degree of iron overload.

Treatment

- Therapeutic phlebotomy is a safe and effective way of decreasing body iron. Guidelines for the initiation of therapeutic phlebotomy proposed by the Hemochromatosis Working Group recommend therapeutic phlebotomy regardless of symptoms in the following patients:
  - Men with serum ferritin levels ≥300 μg/L
  - Women with serum ferritin levels ≥200 μg/L
  - Therapeutic phlebotomy consists of weekly removal of 1 unit of blood until ferritin is decreased to 10 to 20 μg/L and maintenance at 50 μg/L
  - Dietary recommendations: Avoidance of iron supplementation, large quantities of vitamin C, raw seafood.
  - Screening for hemochromatosis: First-degree relatives of patients with HH should be screened with genetic testing for mutations in the *HFE* gene. Iron, total iron-binding capacity, and ferritin levels should be checked in patients over the age of 18 years who are mutation positive.

Autoimmune Hepatitis

Autoimmune hepatitis (AIH) is a chronic inflammatory liver disease of unknown etiology associated with elevated autoantibodies and hypergammaglobulinemia.

Epidemiology/Pathogenesis

- AIH prevalence has been estimated to be ~1.5/100,000.
- Women are more commonly affected than men.
- It is hypothesized that autoimmune hepatitis results from the exposure of an environmental antigen in a genetically predisposed host that triggers an antibody response directed against hepatocyte antigens. The inflammatory response results in necrosis, fibrosis, and cirrhosis of the liver.
- Genetic predisposition: AIH has been associated with HLA class I B8, class II DR3, and DR 52a in whites and HLA DR4 in Asians.
- Environmental triggers: Hepatitis viruses, Epstein–Barr virus, and prior measles infections have been implicated.
- Autoantigens: Sialoglycoprotein receptor has been implicated as a target for cell-mediated immune response seen in AIH. Antibodies to antinuclear, antismooth muscle, and antiactin antibodies in AIH are nonspecific and are not related to the pathogenesis.

TABLE 6-3 Autoantibodies in Autoimmune Hepatitis Overlap Syndrome and Autoimmune Cholangiopathy

Autoimmune Hepatitis	Antinuclear Antibody
Type 1 (classic)	Antismooth muscle antibody Antiactin[a] antibody Antisialo glycoprotein antibody Antimitochondrial antibody (rare)
Type 2	Antiliver kidney microsomal antibody Antiliver cytosol 1
Overlap syndrome	Antimitochondrial antibody
Autoimmune cholangiopathy	Antinuclear antibody

[a]Antiactin antibodies are not clinically tested for but antismooth muscle antibody in concentration >1:320 is suggestive of the presence of antiactin antibodies, which are highly specific for AIH.

- Defective suppressor T-cell function: This theory has been supported by the response to glucocorticoid therapy.

Classification

- AIH is divided into the Classic Type I and Type 2 based on autoantibodies (Table 6-3).
- Overlap syndrome: Patients have clinical and histopathologic features of AIH but autoantibodies seen with primary biliary cirrhosis (antimitochondrial antibodies).
- Autoimmune cholangiopathy: Patients have clinical features of primary biliary cirrhosis and primary sclerosing cholangitis without antimitochondrial antibodies.

Clinical Manifestations

- Patients may be asymptomatic and incidentally diagnosed due to elevated liver function tests.
- Mild nonspecific symptoms fatigue, malaise, anorexia, vague abdominal complaints, or small joint arthralgia.
- Severe liver dysfunction and fulminant hepatic failure with jaundice, coagulopathy, and elevated transaminases that mimic acute viral hepatitis.
- AIH is associated with other autoimmune diseases including autoimmune thyroiditis, Type 1 diabetes, ulcerative colitis (UC), and rheumatoid arthritis.

Diagnosis

- Laboratory tests
  - Elevated globulin levels

- Serology: autoantibodies detailed in Table 6-3.
- Liver biopsy: AIH is characterized by mononuclear cell periportal infiltrate that invades the limiting plate. The periportal infiltrate and consequent piecemeal necrosis spares the biliary tree. In later stages there is bridging fibrosis between the portal tract and the central vein with distortion in lobular architecture.

Treatment

- Initiation of treatment depends on the severity of symptoms and histology, degree of LFT abnormalities, and risk of adverse effects.
- Patients without any symptoms and mild inflammation on liver biopsy may be followed with serial LFTs and biopsy.
- Corticosteroids are the mainstay of therapy. Patients on steroids should be on calcium supplementation for osteoporosis prevention and, depending on the dose and duration of steroids, should be on prophylaxis for *Pneumocystis carinii* pneumonia.
- Azathioprine may be used for steroid-sparing effects. Side effects include bone marrow suppression. Azathioprine, a prodrug, is metabolized to 6-mercaptopurine (active metabolite) (6-MP) and subsequently to 6-methylmercaptopurine (6-MMP), 6-methyl-thioinosine 5′-monophosphate, and 6-thioguanine (6-TG) by the enzyme thiopurine methyltransferase (TPMT). Patients on azathioprine should have TPMT activity tested, as enzyme activity may be lower in patients with certain polymorphisms. In such patients, toxicity can occur with the accumulation of 6-MP.

Complications

AIH, as with all causes of cirrhosis, is associated with an increased risk of primary hepatocellular carcinoma.

Primary Biliary Cirrhosis

Primary biliary cirrhosis (PBC) is characterized by T-cell– mediated destruction of intralobular bile ducts.

Epidemiology/Pathogenesis

- The incidence of PBC has been estimated in studies to be ~2.7 per 100,000 person years.
- Women are affected more often than men with disease onset between the third and sixth decade.
- It is hypothesized that primary biliary cirrhosis results from the exposure of an environmental antigen in a genetically predisposed host that triggers the production of antibody response directed against intralobular bile duct antigens.

- Genetic susceptibility: There is a weak association between PBC and HLA-DR8 and HLA DPB1.
- Environmental trigger: A number of bacteria and viruses have been implicated including *Chlamydia* and *Propionibacterium*.
- Autoantigen: Mitochondrial autoantigens and more specifically the E2 component of pyruvate dehydrogenase complex (PDC-E2) are the most prevalent autoantigens against which antimitochondrial antibodies are directed.

Clinical Manifestations

- Fatigue and pruritus are the two most common clinical features.
- Hyperpigmentation of the skin due to melanin deposition.
- Other clinical features include joint pain, vague right upper quadrant pain, tendon xanthomas from hyperlipidemia, osteoporosis, and osteomalacia.
- Diarrhea and steatorrhea as a consequence of fat malabsorption occurs due to bile acid deficiency.
- Malabsorption results in the deficiency of fat-soluble vitamins (vitamins A, D, E, and K).
- PBC may be associated with other autoimmune diseases such as Sjogren syndrome, celiac disease, rheumatoid arthritis, and scleroderma (CREST).

Diagnosis

- Liver function tests:
  - Elevated alkaline phosphatase.
  - Total and direct bilirubin are elevated in the late stages and carry a poor prognosis.
  - AST and ALT may be normal or slightly elevated.
- Serology:
  - Antimitochondrial antibodies are the hallmark of PBC.
  - Antinuclear antibodies may be elevated in PBC with overlap syndrome with autoimmune hepatitis.
  - Elevated cholesterol, VLDL, LDL, and HDL.
- Liver biopsy: PBC is graded based on histology into the following stages:

  Stage 0: Normal liver
  Stage I: Inflammation confined to the portal areas
  Stage II: Inflammation or fibrosis confined to portal and periportal areas
  Stage III: Bridging fibrosis
  Stage IV: Cirrhosis

- ERCP: Normal or shows narrow caliber ducts and is indicated in patients in whom primary sclerosing cholangitis (PSC) is a consideration.

Treatment

- Ursodeoxycholic acid is the only approved treatment for PBC. It has been shown to delay progression of PBC to end-stage liver disease and improve survival (Poupon et al. *N Engl J Med.* 1994;330:1342).
- Methotrexate and colchicine have been used, but their role in the treatment of PBC remains unclear.
- There is no role for monitoring disease activity with antimitochondrial antibody, which remains elevated despite treatment.

Complications

- Cirrhosis
- Increased risk of hepatocellular carcinoma

Primary Sclerosing Cholangitis

PSC is a chronic, progressive cholestatic disease of the liver characterized by inflammation, fibrosis, and stricturing of both intra- and extrahepatic bile ducts.

Epidemiology/Pathogenesis

- The incidence of PSC is not well known.
- Males are affected more often than females with onset in the fourth decade.
- There is a strong association of ulcerative colitis and PSC. The true prevalence of UC in PSC has been estimated to be ~90% in some studies.
- The etiology of PSC is not known but proposed mechanisms for pathogenesis include the following:
  - Immune dysfunction: Defects in cellular immunity characterized by T cells against bile duct antigens, and humoral immunity, characterized by antismooth muscle antibody, antinuclear antibody and antinuclearcytoplasmic antibody have been implicated in the pathogenesis of PSC.
  - Genetic susceptibility: There is an association between PSC and HLA-B8, DR3, DRW 52a.
  - Environmental antigens: Bacteria from the colonic wall that gain access through the portal circulation (especially given the high prevalence of UC) have been implicated. *Helicobacter* species, α-hemolytic streptococci, have also been associated with PSC.
  - Direct toxicity/ischemia: Hepatic artery chemoembolization with fluorodeoxyuridine results in bile duct injury similar to that seen in PSC. Ischemia or direct toxic injury has therefore been implicated in the pathogenesis of PSC.

Clinical Manifestations

- Patients may be completely asymptomatic and remain undiagnosed for an average of 2 years.
- Fatigue, pruritus from bile salt deposition in the skin, jaundice, weight loss, fever, steatorrhea from impaired bile acid delivery and malabsorption with resultant fat-soluble vitamin deficiency (A, D, E, and K), osteopenia, osteoporosis, and cirrhosis.
- Median survival for symptomatic patients has been estimated to be 8 to 10 years.
- Age, bilirubin, and splenomegaly have been included in the revised Mayo Clinic Model for PSC and are independent predictors of mortality.

Diagnosis

- Liver function tests:
  - Elevated alkaline phosphatase
  - AST and ALT may be elevated (two- to threefold)
  - Increased bilirubin levels fluctuate in PSC and persistent elevations suggest the presence of advanced disease
- Serology: p-ANCA is elevated in 30% to 80% of cases but lack specificity as they can be elevated in AIH, UC, and PBC. Other nonspecific antibodies antinuclear antibody (ANA), anti-smooth muscle antibody (ASMA), antithyroid peroxidase, and rheumatoid factor may be present. Antimitochondrial antibody found in PBC is rarely positive in PSC.
- Imaging of the biliary tree: ERCP, MRCP, or PTC demonstrates characteristic beads-on-string appearance with intrahepatic and extrahepatic biliary ductal saccular dilatation with intervening normal areas
- Liver biopsy:
  - Indicated for assessing disease severity and prognosis.
  - Stage I Portal stage: Nonspecific inflammation confined to the limiting plate around the portal tract
  - Stage II Periportal stage: Inflammation extends beyond the limiting plate with periportal and portal fibrosis
  - Stage III Septal stage: Bridging fibrosis and necrosis
  - Stage IV: Cirrhosis with complete fibrosis and nodular regeneration

Treatment

- Anti-inflammatory and immunomodulatory drugs have been used with no change in natural history of PSC. High-dose ursodeoxycholeic acid protects against bile acid–induced injury and has been shown to improve liver function tests and decrease inflammation.

- ERCP with stenting of dominant stricture. Cholangiocarcinoma should be ruled out with cytology during stricture dilatation.
- Liver transplant is the treatment of choice for advanced PSC.

Complications

- Bacterial cholangitis
- Choledocholithiasis and cholelithiasis from cholesterol/pigment stones
- Cholangiocarcinoma: Patients with PSC have an estimated 10% to 15% lifetime risk.
- Colon cancer: Patients with PSC and UC have an increased risk of colon cancer, which may be related to the exposure of the proximal colon to bile acids. All patients with PSC should undergo flexible sigmoidoscopy with random biopsies to establish a diagnosis of UC. Once concomitant UC has been established, it has been recommended that patients undergo annual colonoscopy with biopsies every 10 cm.

TUMORS OF THE LIVER

Malignant tumors of the liver are more common than benign tumors. The most common malignant tumor is metastatic malignancy.

Hepatocellular Carcinoma

Epidemiology/Pathogenesis

- Hepatocellular carcinoma (HCC) is the fifth most frequent cancer and the third most common cause of cancer death in the world.
- Males are more frequently affected than females and the mean age of presentation varies with demography.
- Risk factors for HCC include the chronic hepatitis C, hepatitis B carrier state, aflatoxin exposure, hemochromatosis, and cirrhosis.
- Chronic HCV infection in patients with cirrhosis is a risk factor for HCC. Genotype 1b may be an independent risk factor for HCC.
- Chronic hepatitis B carrier state carries a higher risk of HCC with exposure in early life. Patients who are HBe Ag positive and those with cirrhosis have a higher risk of HCC. However, unlike hepatitis C, HCC in hepatitis B can occur in patients with or without cirrhosis. HBV DNA levels are an independent predictor of HCC risk.

- Dietary exposure to fungal aflatoxin produced by *Aspergillus flavus* in beans, grain, soil, and decaying vegetables. Aflatoxin once metabolized by the liver may be responsible for mutations in the *p53* tumor suppressor gene.
- Cirrhosis from any cause is associated with an increased risk from HCC.

Clinical Manifestations

- Right upper quadrant pain from capsule stretch by tumor.
- Sudden onset of right upper quadrant pain and hypotension suggests intraperitoneal bleeding from tumor rupture.
- Jaundice from obstruction of bile ducts or tumor infiltration of the liver.
- Weight loss
- Palpable mass
- Fever
- Metastatic disease to the bones, brain, or lung
- Paraneoplastic manifestations include:
  - Hypoglycemia from insulin like growth factor
  - Watery diarrhea in certain cases that can be severe enough to cause hypokalemia
  - Hypercalcemia from parathyroid hormone–related peptide
  - Increased red cell mass from erythropoietin produced by the tumor
  - Cutaneous paraneoplastic manifestations include dermatomyositis, pemphigus foliaceus, sudden appearance of multiple seborrheic keratoses (sign of Leser–Trélat) often in association with acanthosis nigracans, pityriasis rotunda (round hyperpigmented sharply demarcated scaling patches), and porphyria cutanea tarda (development of vesicles and hemorrhagic bullae in patients after minor trauma or exposure to the sun, especially in patients with HCV with HCC).

Diagnosis

The diagnosis of HCC should be suspected in patients with cirrhosis with decompensation, with rising serum AFP (a glycoprotein produced by the fetal liver and yolk sac that is elevated in HCC), or if nodules are seen on screening ultrasound.

- Imaging studies include CT with contrast or contrast magnetic resonance imaging (MRI) can be used to identify HCC.
- The presence of one imaging study that demonstrated hypervascularity in conjunction with an AFP > 400 ng/mL or two imaging studies that demonstrate arterial hypervascularity make the diagnosis of HCC very likely.

- Liver biopsy carries the risk of seeding and is not routinely performed unless it will change management.
- Staging for HCC: Involves a CT of the chest and bone scan to determine if extrahepatic disease is present and two imaging modalities to exclude intravascular invasion of the tumor.

Treatment

- Partial hepatectomy: This is the treatment of choice in patients with tumors that are confined to the liver (< 5cm), no evidence of intravascular tumor invasion, portal hypertension, and preserved liver function.
- Orthotopic liver transplant (OLT): Considered in patients with tumor <5 cm but unresectable disease secondary to hepatic dysfunction or three separate liver lesions <3 cm in the absence of vascular and nodal invasion.
- Radiofrequency ablation (RFA): RFA produces local necrosis of tissue with the use of alternating current. RFA is used in patients with unresectable disease confined to the liver and is most effective in lesions that are <4 cm in diameter.
- Transarterial chemoembolization (TACE): TACE involves chemoembolization through the hepatic artery with a combination of chemotherapeutic agent such as doxorubicin or cisplatin and lipidol to embolize the vessel. TACE is used in patients with unresectable tumors and is used as a bridge to transplant. Side effects of TACE include contrast allergy, nephropathy, bleeding, and abscess formation. Contraindications for TACE include advanced Child C cirrhosis, renal insufficiency (creatinine >1.8), INR > 1.7, and portal vein thrombosis.

LIVER TRANSPLANT

Orthotopic liver transplant is now a treatment option in patients with decompensated cirrhosis, fulminant hepatic failure, and HCC.

Indications for Liver Transplant

- Decompensated cirrhosis from any etiology. Signs of decompensation include hepatic encephalopathy, variceal bleeding, coagulopathy, ascites, jaundice, and hepatorenal syndrome.
- Patients with alcoholic liver disease must be abstinent for greater than 6 months to be listed for transplant.

TABLE 6-4 Child-Turcotte-Pugh Classification

	1 point	2 points	3 points
Ascites	None	Slight	Moderate
Bilirubin (mg/dL)	<2	2–3	>3
Encephalopathy	0	1–2	3–4
Albumin (g/dL)	>3.5	2.8–3.5	<2.8
INR	<1.7	1.8–2.3	>2.3
CTP score	5–6	Childs A	
	7–9	Childs B	
	10–15	Childs C	

- Patients with HCC are eligible for liver transplant if they have a single lesion <5 cm or the number of lesions is less than or equal to three, lesions each of which is ≤3 cm in diameter.
- Patients with fulminant hepatic failure should be listed when they have grade 2 encephalopathy.
- Child–Pugh score, developed to predict outcomes after shunt surgery, is now used to predict the prognosis of patients with cirrhosis of any etiology (Table 6-4).
- The estimated survival of patients with Childs A is 90% at 10 years and the 1-year survival estimates for Childs B and C are 95% and 50%, respectively.
- United Network for Organ Sharing (UNOS) criteria for organ transplant are an estimated 1-year survival of less than 90%, and therefore patients with CTP (Child–Turcotte–Pugh) score > 7 should be referred for liver transplant.
- MELD score:
  - This score, based on INR, bilirubin, and creatinine, is used to estimate short-term mortality in patients with end-stage liver disease.
  - The MELD score is currently used to prioritize candidates for liver transplant.
  - The minimal MELD criteria to be listed for transplant is 10.
  - MELD calculators available online at http://www.unos.org/resources/MeldPeldCalculator.asp?index=98.
  - Evaluation of patients who may be potential candidates for transplant is outlined in Figure 6-10.

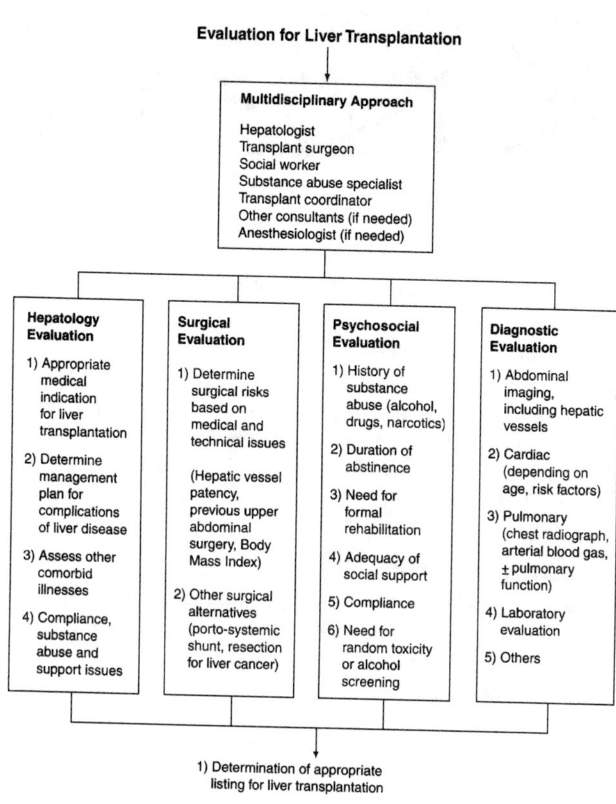

Evaluation for Liver Transplantation
Multidisciplinary Approach
Hepatologist
Transplant surgeon
Social worker
Substance abuse specialist
Transplant coordinator
Other consultants (if needed)
Anesthesiologist (if needed)
Hepatology Evaluation
1) Appropriate medical indication for liver transplantation
2) Determine management plan for complications of liver disease
3) Assess other comorbid illnesses
4) Compliance, substance abuse and support issues
Surgical Evaluation
1) Determine surgical risks based on medical and technical issues
(Hepatic vessel patency, previous upper abdominal surgery, Body Mass Index)
2) Other surgical alternatives (porto-systemic shunt, resection for liver cancer)
Psychosocial Evaluation
1) History of substance abuse (alcohol, drugs, narcotics)
2) Duration of abstinence
3) Need for formal rehabilitation
4) Adequacy of social support
5) Compliance
6) Need for random toxicity or alcohol screening
Diagnostic Evaluation
1) Abdominal imaging, including hepatic vessels
2) Cardiac (depending on age, risk factors)
3) Pulmonary (chest radiograph, arterial blood gas, ± pulmonary function)
4) Laboratory evaluation
5) Others
1) Determination of appropriate listing for liver transplantation
2) Follow-up care plan (medical and substance abuse issues)

Figure 6-10 • Principles in the evaluation of potential candidates for liver transplantation. (From Yamada T, Alpers D, Kaplowitz N, et al. *Textbook of gastroenterology*. Vol. 2. 4th ed. Baltimore: Lippincott Williams & Wilkins; 2003:2478, with permission.)

Chapter 7

Diseases of the Gallbladder and Bile Ducts

Cholelithiasis

Cholelithiasis refers to the presence of stones in the gallbladder.

Epidemiology/Pathogenesis

Biliary colic is caused by the contraction of the gallbladder in response to a fatty meal that results in the obstruction of the cystic duct and resultant pain from increased pressure within the gallbladder. The relaxation of the gallbladder results in release of the stone/sludge obstruction and resolution of pain.

Clinical Manifestations

- Most patients with gallstones are asymptomatic.
- One third of patients with gallstones have symptoms of biliary colic, including epigastric or right upper quadrant pain that radiates to the right shoulder blade. Episodes last 15 min to 3 h.
- Pain may be associated with nausea, vomiting, and diaphoresis.

Physical Examination

- Right upper quadrant tenderness during an attack without guarding, rigidity, or rebound.
- After the resolution of an attack the physical exam is completely normal.

Diagnosis

- Liver function tests are characteristically normal.
- Abdominal ultrasound: An inexpensive test to image the gallbladder. Stones in the gallbladder produce a characteristic echogenic focus with an acoustic shadow.

Treatment

- Asymptomatic patients with incidental gallstones do not need to be treated.
- Patients with symptomatic gallstones or complications, who are surgical candidates, should undergo cholecystectomy.

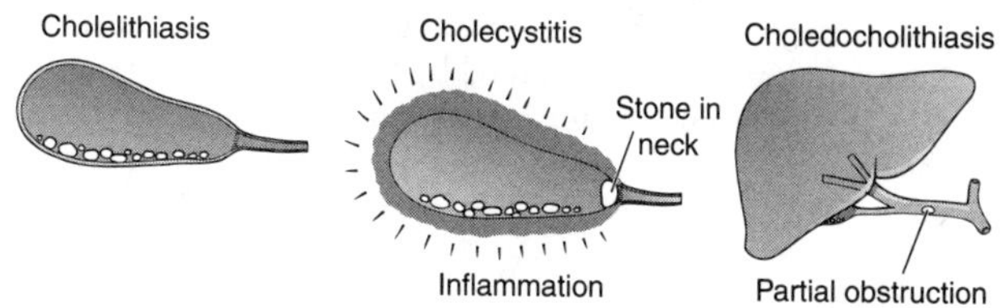

Figure 7-1 • Biliary pathology. (From Karp S, Morris J, Soybel D. *Blueprints surgery.* 3rd ed. Oxford: Blackwell; 2004, with permission.)

- Patients with symptomatic gallstones, who are not operative candidates, may be treated with ursodeoxycholeic acid with or without ERCP with sphincterotomy.

Acute Calculous Cholecystitis

Etiology/Pathogenesis

Persistent obstruction of the cystic duct by a gallstone or sludge results in inflammation of the gallbladder.

Clinical Manifestations

- Right upper quadrant pain with radiation to the interscapular region or the right shoulder blade.
- Associated with nausea and vomiting.
- Fever.
- Patients often have a history of biliary colic in the past.

Physical Examination

Murphy's sign: Abrupt cessation of inspiration secondary to pain on palpation of the right upper quadrant.

Diagnosis

- Acute cholecystitis should be suspected in patients with right upper quadrant pain, fever, and leukocytosis.
- Elevated white cell count.
- Normal liver function tests in uncomplicated cholecystitis.
- Abdominal ultrasound (USG): This is a sensitive (85% to 90%) and specific (70% to 100%) imaging modality for acute cholecystitis. Diagnostic criteria for acute cholecystitis include cholelithiasis, a sonographic Murphy's sign with tenderness over the sonographically localized gallbladder, pericholecystic fluid, wall edema, or thickening greater than 3 mm, and gallbladder dilatation.
- Hepatobiliary imaging with technetium-99m-labeled hepatic iminodiacetic acid (HIDA): This nuclear test is as sensitive as

ultrasonography for biliary pathology. Iminodiacetic acid is injected intravenously, absorbed by the liver, excreted into the bile, and then concentrated in the gallbladder. Failure to visualize the gallbladder implies cystic duct obstruction as seen in acute cholecystitis secondary to edema or from obstruction due to a gallstone.

Treatment

- Patients with acute cholecystitis should be hospitalized.
- Antibiotic treatment should include coverage for *Enterococcus* and enteric Gram-negative rods. Ampicillin and gentamicin can be used to treat patients with cholecystitis empirically.
- Patients that are low risk for cholecystectomy should undergo surgery following a few days of antibiotics.
- Patients who are at high risk for surgery and cannot be treated definitively with surgery should be considered for ursodeoxycholeic acid treatment for gallstone dissolution.
- All patients who clinically deteriorate should undergo percutaneous cholecystostomy drainage to decompress the gallbladder.

Complications

- Gangrene of the gallbladder is the most frequent complication.
- Emphysematous gallbladder is caused by infection with gas-forming organisms, e.g., *Clostridium welchii* and enteric Gram-negative rods.
- Perforation can occur in patients with gangrene and may not produce classic symptoms in the elderly individuals and in patients with diabetes
- Cholecystoenteric fistula from perforation of the bowel wall
- Gallstone ileus from small bowel obstruction by a gallstone that has entered the lumen via a cholecystoenteric fistula
- Pericholecystic abscess secondary to perforation

Differential Diagnosis

- Biliary colic, cholangitis, choledocholithiasis, and acute hepatitis

Acute Acalculous Cholecystitis

Etiology/Pathogenesis

- Inflammation of the gallbladder that occurs in the absence of gallstones.
- Acalculous cholecystitis accounts for 10% cases of acute cholecystitis.
- Predisposing condition are hypotension; mechanical ventilation with high positive end expiratory pressure (PEEP) has been

postulated to decrease portal pressure resulting in ischemic injury, total parenteral nutrition, diabetes, and infections.
- Once acalculous cholecystitis develops, patients have a high incidence of secondary infections of the gallbladder.

Clinical Manifestations

- Patients are predominately male and older than 50 years.
- Presentation is similar to patients with acute cholecystitis with right upper quadrant pain with radiation to the interscapular region or the right shoulder blade.
- Nausea, vomiting.
- Fever.
- Jaundice from common bile duct (CBD) obstruction due to inflammation around the cystic duct and consequent elevations in liver function tests (LFTs) can be seen in acalculous cholecystitis but are not seen with calculous cholecystitis.

Physical Examination

- Right upper quadrant mass may be palpable unlike in patients with acute calculous cholecystitis.
- Unlike calculous cholecystitis, icterus may be present.

Diagnosis

- Elevated white cell count.
- LFTs may be mildly elevated from CBD obstruction from inflammation around the cystic duct with mildly elevated transaminses, bilirubin, and alkaline phosphatase.
- Abdominal USG: Characteristic gallbladder wall thickening (>4 mm) or edema, intramural gas, sloughed gallbladder mucosa, pericholecystic fluid, sonographic Murphy's sign, or failure to visualize the gallbladder.
- Abdominal computed tomography (CT) scan is as sensitive as an abdominal USG and has the advantage of having the ability to rule out other intra-abdominal pathology.

Treatment

- Broad-spectrum antibiotics to cover enteric Gram-negative rods and anaerobes.
- Definitive treatment is with percutaneous or open cholecystostomy.

Complications

Acalculous cholecystitis is associated with the same complications as calculous cholecystitis listed previously, but they may develop more rapidly.

Differential Diagnosis

- Biliary colic, cholangitis, choledocholithiasis, and acute hepatitis.

Chronic Cholecystitis

Following recurrent episodes of acute cholecystitis or colic, the gallbladder becomes chronically thickened and fibrotic. Patients have few clinical symptoms and usually present only with complications of gallstones. Intramural calcification of the gallbladder (porcelain gallbladder) is a rare manifestation of chronic cholecystitis. Although patients are asymptomatic, porcelain gallbladder is a premalignant condition and therefore an indication for cholecystectomy.

Choledocholithiasis

Choledocholithiasis is defined as the presence of stones in the CBD.

Epidemiology/Pathogenesis

- Most CBD stones arise in the gallbladder and migrate into the CBD. However, some pigment stones can form in the CBD itself.
- Risk factors for the development of CBD stones include those that increase the concentration of unconjugated bilirubin (hemolysis or bacterial beta-glucoronidase that deconjugates bilirubin in the bile ducts) or increase stasis in the bile ducts (sphincter of Oddi dysfunction, diverticulae, and stenosis).

Clinical Manifestations

Patients are rarely asymptomatic and usually present with right upper quadrant or epigastric pain that radiates to the back or right shoulder blade.

Diagnosis

- Elevated transaminases that are released immediately due to hepatic injury; alkaline phosphatase is later elevated. Total bilirubin and increased direct bilirubin is elevated due to duct obstruction.
- Abdominal USG demonstrates dilatation of the CBD above the level of the stone.

Treatment

- Endoscopic retrograde cholangiopancreatogram (ERCP) with stone extraction and sphicterotomy is the procedure of choice.
- Magnetic resonance cholangiopancreatogram (MRCP) is reserved only for cases where the index of suspicion is low as, unlike ERCP, it is only of diagnostic value and is not therapeutic.

Complications

- Acute cholangitis
- Gallstone pancreatitis

Differential Diagnosis

- Biliary colic, cholangitis, choledocholithiasis, acute cholecystitis, and acute hepatitis.

Acute Cholangitis

Infection of the biliary tree characterized by the triad of fever, jaundice, and right upper quadrant pain.

Epidemiology/Pathogenesis

- Acute cholangitis is caused by bacterial infection of the biliary tract in the setting of a partial CBD obstruction by stones/ stricture resulting in increased intrabiliary pressure and the transmigration of bacteria from portal circulation.
- Acute cholangitis can also occur when the sphincter of Oddi, which acts as a barrier to the bowel flora, is disrupted by a sphincterotomy or stent.

Clinical Manifestations

- Charcot's triad:
  - Fever
  - Right upper quadrant pain
  - Jaundice
- Reynolds pentad:
  - Fever
  - Right upper quadrant pain
  - Jaundice
  - Hypotension
  - Altered mental status

Diagnosis

- Laboratory tests:
  - Elevated alkaline phosphatase
  - Elevated total bilirubin
  - Elevated direct bilirubin
  - Elevated transaminases
  - Elevated white cell count with left shift
- Right upper quadrant ultrasound: May reveal CBD stone and CBD dilatation. However, small stones may be missed on ultrasound and in the early stages ductal dilatation may not be seen.
- ERCP: This is the procedure of choice as it is both diagnostic and therapeutic.

Treatment

- Intravenous fluids
- Broad-spectrum antibiotics: Once blood cultures have been obtained, antibiotics should be initiated to cover *Enterococcus, Escherichia coli*, and *Klebsiella*. Ampicillin and gentamicin or a fluoroquinolone such as levofloxacin may be used.
- Biliary decompression: ERCP with stone removal and sphincterotomy is the procedure of choice. If it is unsuccessful, open or percutaneous cholecystostomy may be performed.

Differential Diagnosis

- Cholecystitis, Mirizzi syndrome, and infected choledochal cyst

Cystic Disease of the Gallbladder

Choledochal cysts are cystic dilatation of the biliary tree and more specifically the CBD.

Epidemiology/Pathogenesis

- Choledochal cysts are rare, with 4,000 cases reported worldwide (Fig. 7-2).
- Pathogenesis of choledochal cysts remains unclear; proposed etiologies have included weakness of the ductal wall and distal duct obstruction.
- Type I disease is the most frequently seen.
- Type V disease is characterized by intrahepatic bile duct dilatation and is called Caroli disease. Caroli syndrome is defined as intrahepatic bile duct dilatation associated with congenital hepatic fibrosis.
- Stasis of bile in dilated bile ducts results in stone formation and partial duct obstruction with bacteremia, which results in recurrent episodes of cholangitis.

Clinical Manifestations

- Manifest in childhood with pain, jaundice, and palpable abdominal mass.
- Patients may present with recurrent episodes of cholangitis or hepatic abscesses.
- In rare cases patients may present with cirrhosis and portal hypertension.

Diagnosis

- Abdominal USG
- MRCP

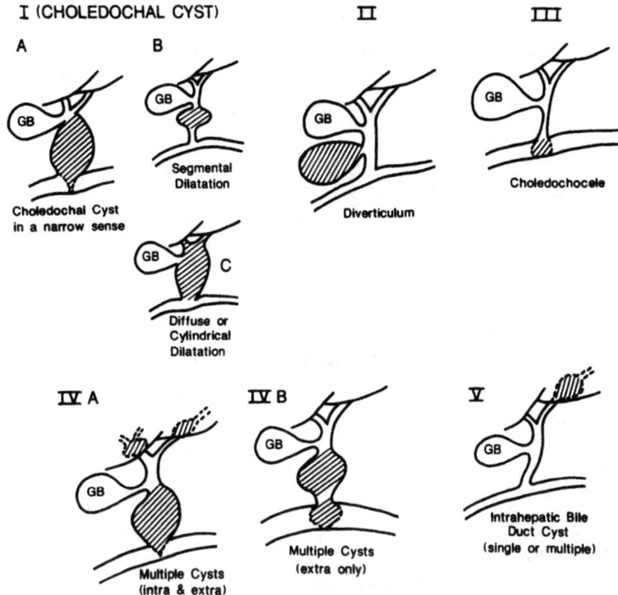

Figure 7-2 • Todani's classification of biliary cysts based on location. Hatched areas represent cystic dilations. (From Yamada T, Alpers D, Kaplowitz N, et al. *Textbook of gastroenterology*. Vol. 2. 4th ed. Baltimore: Lippincott Williams & Wilkins; 2003:2226, with permission).

- ERCP, which may be of particular utility in the diagnosis of Type III disease with choledochocele

Treatment

- ERCP with sphincterotomy is used to extract intraductal stones that are extrahepatic.
- Definitive treatment is cyst excision and if possible with cholecystectomy at the time of cyst excision.
- In patients with Caroli syndrome, hepatic resection for localized disease or hepaticojejunostomy for extensive disease, or liver transplant are options.

Cholangiocarcinoma

Carcinoma of the epithelium lining the intrahepatic or extrahepatic biliary tree. Cholangiocarcinoma is predominantly adenocarcinoma (90%) followed by squamous cell carcinoma (10%).

Epidemiology/Pathogenesis

- Cholangiocarcinomas are rare, with an incidence of 1 to 2 per 100,000 population
- Risk factors for cholangiocarcinoma include:
  - Choledochal cysts
  - Primary sclerosing cholangitis
  - Ulcerative colitis
  - *Chlornorchis sinensis* infection
  - Hereditary nonpolyposis colorectal cancer
  - Toxin exposure (e.g., thorotrast)

Clinical Features

- Obstructive jaundice with icterus, dark urine, clay-colored stool, and pruritis
- Right upper quadrant pain
- Weight loss
- Fever

Diagnosis

- Laboratory tests:
  - Elevated alkaline phosphatase
  - Elevated total and direct bilirubin
  - Elevated transaminases with liver injury from longstanding obstruction
- Abdominal USG may reveal an intraductal mass with ductal dilatation
- Abdominal CT scan can visualize tumor, ductal dilatation, associated adenopathy, and metastatic disease.
- MRCP may be superior to CT in imaging cholangiocarcinoma, without exposure to contrast.
- ERCP has the advantage of being able to collect cytologic brushings to confirm the diagnosis and provide stenting if necessary.

Treatment

- Definitive treatment is with surgery. Lesions are potentially resectable if there is no vascular or local invasion, liver or distant metastatic disease, or adenopathy.
- Distal lesions are treated with pancreaticoduodenectomy (Whipple procedure), intrahepatic lesions are treated with hepatic resection, and perihilar tumors are treated with resection of the extrahepatic bile ducts, gallbladder, and hepatic lobectomy with Roux-en-Y hepaticojejunostomy.
- Local recurrence is common after surgery and adjuvant therapy with radiation or chemoradiation (mitomycin and 5-fluorouracil) have been proposed.

- For patients with unresectable disease (60% to 90% of patients at presentation), palliative stenting or biliary enteric bypass can be performed with or without postoperative radiation. The role of chemotherapy in such patients is controversial.

Carcinoma of the Gallbladder

Epidemiology/Pathogenesis

- Gallbladder cancer is a rare malignancy and has a high associated mortality due to the late stage at the time of diagnosis.
- Gallbladder cancers are predominantly adenocarcinomas followed by squamous cell carcinoma, small cell carcinoma, and lymphoma.
- Risk factors for gallbladder cancer include the following:
  - Gallstones, with increased risk associated with an increase in size of gallstones
  - Porcelain gallbladder
  - Gallbladder polyps
  - Congenital cysts of the biliary tract

Clinical Manifestations

- Right upper quadrant pain
- Weight loss
- Anorexia, malaise
- In rare cases, patients may present with obstructive jaundice due to tumor invasion of the porta hepatis.

Diagnosis

- Abdominal USG may demonstrate thickening of the gallbladder wall or a mass.
- Abdominal CT scan can better define gallbladder mass, involvement of the liver and lymph nodes. However, it is not possible to distinguish benign from malignant polyps.
- Endoscopic ultrasound can be used to determine lymph node involvement, depth of tumor invasion, and distinguish benign from malignant polyps.

Treatment

- Definitive treatment is surgical resection. Candidates for surgery include those without invasion or encasement of vascular structures, ascites, hepatic, or intraperitoneal metastatic disease.
- Surgical options include simple cholecystectomy or radical cholecystectomy depending on the tumor stage.

- Adjuvant chemoradiation (mitomycin and 5-fluorouracil) have been used to decrease local recurrence rate but have not been shown to have a mortality benefit.
- In patients with unresectable disease the benefit of chemotherapy, with gemcitabine, and 5-fluorouracil, cisplatin, or capcitabine, over supportive care has not been established.

Chapter

8 Diseases of the Pancreas

Acute Pancreatitis

Acute pancreatitis is characterized by inflammation of the pancreas that results in severe, acute onset of abdominal pain and elevated pancreatic enzymes.

Epidemiology/Pathogenesis

Acute pancreatitis is a common disorder and affects 1 to 2 per 10,000 individuals per year.

Risk Factors

- Toxins and drugs
  - Alcohol by direct and indirect toxic effects, sphincter of Oddi dysfunction, and production of proteinaceous plugs in pancreatic secretion that obstruct the pancreatic duct can result in pancreatitis.
  - Medications: Azathioprine, alpha methyl dopa, metronidazole, nitrofurantoin, mercaptopurine, valproic acid, and erythromycin have all been associated with acute pancreatitis.
  - Scorpion bite: *Tityus trinitatis* venom causes the release of pancreatic enzymes and sphincter of Oddi spasm.
- Obstruction
  - Gallstones: It has been proposed that gallstones cause obstruction of the ampulla of Vater and the reflux of bile into the pancreatic duct or obstruct the pancreatic duct thereby precipitating pancreatitis.
  - Pancreas divisum: This is a congenital abnormality in which the ventral pancreatic duct that drains into the major papilla (duct of Wirsung) does not fuse with the dorsal pancreatic duct (duct of Santorini), which normally drains into the minor papillae. Failure of fusion of the two ducts results in the dorsal duct draining most of the pancreas into the minor papilla. It has been suggested that resistance to the flow of pancreatic secretions through the duct of Santorini and consequent increased pancreatic ductal pressure result in pancreatitis. Pancreas divisum has been associated with recurrent pancreatitis.
  - Pancreatic tumors
  - Sphincter of Oddi dysfunction

- Metabolic abnormalities
  - Hypertriglyceridemia: Levels >1000 mg/dL have been associated with pancreatitis. The release of toxic free fatty acids secondary to the action of pancreatic lipase on triglycerides results in damage to pancreatic blood vessels.
  - Hypercalcemia
- Trauma
  - Blunt trauma to the abdomen
  - Post-endoscopic retrograde cholangiopancreatogram (ERCP), postoperative
- Vascular abnormalities
  - Hypotension
  - Vasculitis
  - Emboli
- Infections
  - Parasitic: *Chlororchis sinensis* and *Ascaris lumbricoides*
  - Bacterial: *Mycobacterium tuberculosis, M. avium* complex, *Mycoplasma, Legionella,* and *Campylobacter*
  - Viral: Hepatitis A, B, mumps, adenovirus, cytomegalovirus (CMV), Epstein–Barr virus, HIV, and Coxsackie
- Triggered by one of the above insults, inactive pancreatic zymogens are converted into active and proinflammatory mediators are released.

Clinical Manifestations

Patients present with sudden onset of epigastric pain that radiates to the back.

Diagnosis

- Laboratory features
  - Elevated amylase is sensitive for acute pancreatitis but not specific as it is produced by the other organs, including the salivary gland, lung, and fallopian tube. Amylase levels tend to be lower in patients with alcoholic pancreatitis than other forms. Amylase levels may be artificially elevated in patients with renal failure.
  - Elevated lipase is a more sensitive and specific test for acute pancreatitis than amylase. Similar to amylase, lipase is a useful early marker for pancreatitis but remains elevated longer than amylase.
  - The degree of elevation of amylase or lipase is not an indicator of disease severity and is not of prognostic value.
  - Elevated transaminases and more specifically ALT are suggestive of gallstone pancreatitis as the etiology.
  - Elevated bilirubin may also be seen transiently in patients with gallstone pancreatitis.
- Abdominal ultrasound (USG)
  - Useful in visualizing the biliary tree to determine if gallstones precipitated pancreatitis.

- Computed tomography (CT) abdomen: Abdominal CT is the imaging modality of choice to confirm the diagnosis of pancreatitis, determine the extent, and in ruling out other intra-abdominal pathology. If the diagnosis of pancreatitis is not in doubt, a CT scan can be avoided in the first 24 h as it may take up to 48 h for pancreatic necrosis to be evident.

Prognosis

- The Ranson criteria and the Modified Glasgow Scale are the most commonly used prognostic scores to distinguish mild from severe pancreatitis within the first 48 h after admission (Table 8-1).
- The Acute Physiology and Chronic Health Evaluation (APACHE) II score is based on 12 physiologic variables, the patient's underlying disease, and chronic health. The APACHE II score has the advantage of the ability to predict mortality even after 48 h of admission.
- Hemoconcentration: A hematocrit (HCT) > 44 and failure of the hematocrit to fall by 24 h have been shown to be predictors of necrotizing pancreatitis and multiorgan failure.

Complications

- One fourth of all cases of pancreatitis result in complications and have a mortality of ~10%
- The complications and management of these complications are listed in Table 8-2.

TABLE 8-1 Ranson and Simplified Glasgow Prognostic Scoring Criteria

Ranson	Simplified Glasgow
On admission	Within 48 h
Age > 55 y	Age > 55 y
WBC > 16,000 mm^3	WBC > 15,000 mm^3
LDH > 350 IU/L	LDH > 600 IU/L
Glucose > 200 IU/L	Glucose > 180 mg/dL
Within 48 h	Albumin < 3.2 g/dL
HCT decrease by > 10%	Calcium < 8 mg/dL
Serum calcium < 8 mg/dL	Arterial PO_2 < 60 mm Hg
Arterial PO_2 < 60 mm Hg	Urea > 45 mg/dL
Base deficit > 4 mEq/L	
Estimated fluid sequestration > 6 L	

Adapted from Agarwal N, Pitchumoni CS. Assessment of severity in acute pancreatitis. *Am J Gastroenterol.* 1990;85:356; and Marshall JB. Acute pancreatitis: a review with an emphasis on new developments. *Arch Intern Med.* 1993;153:1185, with permission.

TABLE 8-2 Complications of Acute Pancreatitis

Complication	Cause	Therapy
Local		
Necrosis		
Sterile tissue	Microvascular hypoperfusion	Observation, debridement
Infected tissue	Superimposed bacterial infection	Antibiotics, debridement
Pancreatic-fluid collections		
Pseudocysts	Extravasation of fluid, inflammatory debris in peripancreatic spaces	Observation, drainage
Abscesses	Superimposed bacterial infection	Drainage
Necrotizing obstruction or fistulization of colon	Extension of pancreatic necrosis into adjacent bowel	Observation, surgery
Gastrointestinal hemorrhage		
Ulceration	Stress, ischemia	Transfusions, H2 blockers
Gastric varices	Splenic-vein obstruction	Sclerotherapy, surgery
Rupture of pseudoaneurysm	Digestion of pancreatic blood vessels	Embolization, surgery
Right-sided hydronephrosis	Peripancreatic inflammation in perirenal space	Observation
Splenic rupture or hematoma	Extension of inflammatory process into spleen	Observation, surgery
Systemic		
Shock	Sequestration of retroperitoneal fluid or hemorrhage, kinin activation	Volume replacement, dopamine
Coagulopathy	Circulating process	Fresh-frozen plasma, supportive therapy
Respiratory failure	Release of phospholipase A_2 leading to surfactant degradation	Mechanical ventilation
Acute renal failure	Acute tubular necrosis	Dialysis
Hyperglycemia	Decreased insulin levels, excessive glucagons release	Insulin replacement
Hypocalcemia	Hypoalbuminemia, peripancreatic-fat necrosis	Calcium replacement

(*Continued*)

TABLE 8-2 Complications of Acute Pancreatitis (*Continued*)

Complication	Cause	Therapy
Subcutaneous nodules	Metastatic-fat necrosis	None
Retinopathy	Retinal arteriolar obstruction	None
Psychosis	Demyelination, cerebral hypoperfusion	None

From Steinberg W, Tenner S. Acute pancreatitis. *N Engl J Med*. 1994;330:1198–1210, with permission.

Treatment

- Nil per oral (NPO)
- Close monitoring with measurement of fluid intake and output, blood pressure, and oxygen saturation.
- Aggressive intravenous hydration to ensure HCT < 44%. Fluid resuscitation has not been shown to prevent pancreatic necrosis, but all patients with persistent hemoconcentration at 24 h developed necrotizing pancreatitis (Brown et al. *Pancreatology*. 2002;2(2):104–107).
- Electrolyte monitoring and repletion.
- Pain control and antiemetics.
- Nasogastric tube decompression in patients with severe pancreatitis with persistent emesis and ileus.
- ERCP with sphincterotomy within 24 h of admission has been shown to decrease the incidence of biliary sepsis in patients with gallstone pancreatitis (Fan S-T et al. *N Engl J Med*. 1993; 328:228–232).
- Prophylactic imipenem has been shown to decrease the incidence of pancreatic sepsis in patients with necrotizing pancreatitis.
- Debridement of sterile necrotic pancreatic tissue is controversial. Surgical debridement is warranted in patients with infected pancreatic necrosis.
- Patients with mild disease who improve can resume oral intake. Patients with more severe disease may need nutritional support. There are no data to demonstrate benefit in the use of total parenteral nutrition. Enteral feeding beyond the jejunum, thereby avoiding pancreatic stimulation, has been found to be safe and well tolerated.

Chronic Pancreatitis

Chronic pancreatitis is an inflammatory condition of the pancreas characterized by necrosis and edema superimposed on pre-existing fibrosis and loss of exocrine tissue.

Epidemiology/Pathogenesis

- Prevalence of chronic pancreatitis has been estimated to be 0.04% to 5%.
- Acute pancreatitis does not lead to chronic pancreatitis unless complications of pancreatitis such as pseudocysts or strictures of the pancreatic duct are present.

Risk Factors

- Alcohol use: Accounts for 80% of cases of chronic pancreatitis. The exact pathogenesis is unclear, but it appears to be related to the duration and mean daily alcohol consumed.
- Tropical pancreatitis: Seen in children in India, Southeast Asia, and tropical Africa. Tropical pancreatitis is believed to be associated with protein deficiency or toxins in consumed cassava. Patients present with abdominal pain and a few years later manifest with brittle diabetes.
- Pancreas divisum: Failure of the ventral and dorsal pancreatic ducts to fuse results in the drainage of pancreatic juice through the minor papilla and functional obstruction.
- Pancreatic duct obstruction: Tumor, stenosis, or strictures can result in chronic pancreatitis. Resultant fibrosis can regress if obstruction is relieved.
- Autoimmune pancreatitis: This is characterized by the presence of elevated immunoglobulin G (IgG) levels and several autoantibodies. Patients present with recurrent episodes of mild pancreatitis and may have associated obstructive jaundice due to ductal obstruction around the pancreatic duct caused by the inflamed pancreas. CT shows characteristic sausage appearance of the pancreas and ERCP shows segmental or diffuse narrowing of the pancreatic duct with stenosis of the common bile duct. Treatment with steroids produces a dramatic response.
- Hyperparathyroidism: Chronic hypercalcemia from hyperparathyroidism results in an increase in calcium in pancreatic secretions resulting in calcification and chronic pancreatitis.
- Trauma: Unrecognized trauma can result in ductal disruption. In such cases chronic pancreatitis improves with surgical correction.
- Hereditary pancreatitis: Autosomal dominant inheritance with 80% penetrance. Hereditary pancreatitis is associated with an increased risk of pancreatic cancer.

- Idiopathic pancreatitis: Cystic fibrosis transmembrane conductance regulator mutations have been found in patients previously thought to have idiopathic chronic pancreatitis even though they had no clinical manifestations of cystic fibrosis. The significance of these mutations remains unknown.

Clinical Manifestations

- Epigastric abdominal pain with radiation to the back is characteristic. Pain is aggravated by meals and may exhibit postural variation with worsening in the supine position and relief with sitting up or leaning forward.
- Pain is often associated with nausea and vomiting.
- Weight loss may be significant and is seen due to a decrease in intake secondary to pain.
- Steatorrhea and diarrhea result from pancreatic enzyme deficiency. These symptoms occur when secretion is reduced to 10% and are therefore seen late in the course of the disease.
- Diabetes due to deficiency in insulin production results late in the course of the disease.

Physical Examination

- Epigastric tenderness
- Fever or an epigastric mass is suggestive of a pseudocyst.

Diagnosis

- Plain radiograph abdomen: Pancreatic calcification may be seen in one third of cases.
- Abdominal CT scan: Shows pancreatic calcification, ductal dilatation, edema of the pancreas, and pseudocysts.
- Laboratory tests
  - Amylase and lipase may be completely normal or only mildly elevated due the inability of the fibrotic pancreas to synthesize these enzymes.
  - Aspartate transaminases (AST) and alanine aminotransferase (ALT) may be elevated in patients secondary to alcoholic liver disease.
  - In rare cases serum bilirubin and alkaline phosphatase may be elevated due to compression of the intrapancreatic bile duct from pancreatic edema.
- ERCP: Diagnostic and therapeutic procedure of choice; demonstrates characteristic beaded appearance of the main pancreatic duct and ectatic branches.
- Pancreatic exocrine function tests: These tests are warranted if, despite normal ERCP results, there is high suspicion for chronic pancreatitis. Secretin stimulation test is the gold standard and

involves the measurement of duodenal bicarbonate in response to the administration of secretin. Levels less than 80 mEq/L are suggestive of chronic pancreatitis.

Treatment

- Pain control with analgesics.
- Patients with continued pain should undergo ERCP to define the pancreatic duct size and morphology. In patients with dilated ducts, decompression with internal surgical drainage or pancreaticojejunostomy (Puestow procedure) or stent placement. Pancreatic resection has been tried in patients with nondilated ducts.
- Malabsorption is treated with pancreatic enzymes.
- Pancreatic pseudocysts merit drainage if they are symptomatic or persist for 6 weeks. Drainage can be performed internally via surgery with a cystogastrostomy, cystojejunostomy, or Roux-en-Y cystojejunostomy or endoscopically with the creation of a cystoenteric fistula. External drainage is complicated by the formation of a fistula and infection.
- Duodenal or biliary obstruction by a pseudocyst or from fibrosis can be treated with cyst decompression, gastrojejunostomy, choledochoenterotomy or endoscopically with the placement of a stent.
- Pancreatic ascites from ductal disruption is treated with distal pancreatectomy or Roux-en-Y of the jejunum to the disrupted pancreatic duct.

Complications

Pseudocyst, pancreatic ascites, obstructive jaundice, duodenal obstruction, or splenic vein thrombosis.

Differential Diagnosis

Acute pancreatitis, pancreatic cancer, mesenteric ischemia, and peptic ulcer disease

Pancreatic Cancer

Epidemiology/Pathogenesis

- Pancreatic cancer has been estimated to be the fourth most common cancer in men and fifth most common in women.
- Peak incidence is in the seventh decade with male preponderance.
- 90% of pancreatic cancers are ductal adenocarcinomas. The rest are acinar cell carcinoma, lymphomas, and sarcomas.
- Two thirds of pancreatic cancers are located in the head of the pancreas.

Risk Factors

- Cigarette smoking has been strongly associated with pancreatic cancer with a relative risk of 2 of pancreatic cancer among smokers and a decrease in risk with cessation.
- Genetic factors: Hereditary nonpolyposis colorectal cancer (HNPCC), familial atypical multiple mole melanoma (FAMMM), Von Hippel Lindau (VHL), familial adenomatous polyposis (FAP), Peutz-Jeghers, and multiple endocrine neoplasia (MEN 1) all carry an increased risk of pancreatic cancer.
- Pancreatitis: Secondary to chronic inflammation, is associated with an increased risk of pancreatic cancer.

Clinical Manifestations

- Pain is usually epigastric and may radiate to the back.
- Significant weight loss with loss of >10% weight in 6 months.
- Obstructive jaundice due to tumor compression of the common bile duct with pruritus, icterus, dark urine, and clay-colored stool.
- Duodenal and gastric outlet obstruction resulting in associated nausea and vomiting.
- Superficial thrombophlebitis.

Physical Examination

- Pancreatic mass or enlarged gallbladder may be palpable.
- Scleral icterus.
- Left supraclavicular lymph node (Virchow node).

Diagnosis

- Laboratory tests
- Abdominal ultrasound may show dilated bile ducts and a mass at the head of the pancreas but is of limited sensitivity.
- Abdominal CT scan has higher sensitivity in detecting pancreatic mass and can determine the extent of metastatic disease.
- ERCP has high sensitivity and specificity for pancreatic cancer and is indicated in cases when CT does not reveal a mass lesion and stricturing of the pancreatic duct is present. Double-duct sign (stricture of the pancreatic and common bile duct) and pancreatic duct stricture >1 cm are suggestive of malignancy.
- Endoscopic ultrasound (EUS) is more accurate than an abdominal CT scan in determining tumor staging and vascular invasion of pancreatic tumors. EUS-guided USG is also been used for tissue diagnosis of pancreatic cancer.
- Serum markers: CA 19-9, a tumor marker, has a sensitivity of 80% and specificity of 90% for pancreatic cancer but may be elevated in patients with jaundice without pancreatic cancer (Table 8-3).

TABLE 8-3 Staging of Pancreatic Exocrine Cancer

Definition of TNM

Primary tumor (T)

TX Primary tumor cannot be assessed
T0 No evidence of primary tumor
Tis *In situ* carcinoma
T1 Tumor limited to the pancreas, 2 cm or less in greatest dimension
T2 Tumor limited to the pancreas, more than 2 cm in greatest dimension
T3 Tumor extends beyond the pancreas but without involvement of the celiac axis or the superior mesenteric artery
T4 Tumor involves the celiac axis or the superior mesenteric artery (unresectable primary tumor)

Regional lymph nodes (N)

NX Regional lymph nodes cannot be assessed
N0 No regional lymph node metastasis
N1 Regional lymph node metastasis

Distant metastasis (M)

MX Distant metastasis cannot be assessed
M0 No distant metastasis
M1 Distant metastasis

Stage Grouping

Stage 0	Tis N0 M0
Stage IA	T1 N0 M0
Stage IB	T2 N0 M0
Stage IIA	T3 N0 M0
Stage IIB	T1–3 N1 M0
Stage III	T4 Any N M0
Stage IV	Any T Any N M1

From the American Joint Committee on Cancer (AJCC), Chicago, with permission. The original source for this material is the *AJCC cancer staging manual*. 6th ed. New York: Springer-Verlag; 2002.

Treatment

- Surgical resection: In patients without vascular involvement Whipple procedure consisting of cholecystectomy, partial gastrectomy, and resection of the distal common bile duct, head of the pancreas, duodenum, proximal jejunum, and regional lymph nodes.
- Adjuvant chemoradiation is controversial following resection.
- Palliative therapy: In patients with unresectable pancreatic cancer and in patients with recurrence, relief of biliary obstruction with ERCP and stent placement or surgically with

choledochojejunostomy or cholecystojejunostomy. Duodenal obstruction can be relieved with gastrojejunostomy.
- Pain control with celiac plexus block.
- Pancreatic enzymes may decrease the extent of malabsorption.

Prognosis

- The prognosis of patients with pancreatic cancer depends on the degree of tumor differentiation and the extent of tumor.
- Median survival is 3 to 6 months in patients with metastatic disease and 9 to 12 months for those with locally advanced unresectable disease. The 5-year survival after surgery in patients with resectable disease is approximately 15% to 20%.

Appendix

A Review Questions and Answers

1. A previously healthy 35-year-old man presents to his primary care physician's office with 6 weeks of epigastric pain and retrosternal burning that is exacerbated by meals. He denies any weight loss or change in bowel habits. He remains a nonsmoker, is not on any medications. What is the most appropriate management strategy at this time?

   a. 24-h pH probe
   b. Barium swallow
   c. Upper endoscopy to confirm the diagnosis and rule out Barrett's esophagus and prescribe empiric acid suppression therapy
   d. Prescribe empiric acid suppression therapy
   e. Antireflux surgery

2. A 62-year-old woman with a history of osteoporosis, hypertension, diabetes, atrial fibrillation, and coronary artery disease presents with 6 weeks of epigastric pain that is worse after meals. She is on aspirin, clopidogrel, warfarin, atenolol, and metformin. Physical exam is remarkable for mild epigastric tenderness and rectal exam is heme negative. Laboratory data are unremarkable. What is the most appropriate next step in the management of this patient?

   a. Prescribe empiric acid suppression therapy
   b. Discontinue aspirin therapy
   c. Prescribe misoprostol and continue all current medications
   d. Upper endoscopy and biopsy

3. A 65-year-old man with osteoporosis, hypertension, atrial fibrillation, GERD (gastroesophageal reflux disease), and diabetes presents with dysphagia to solids for 6 weeks and 6-lb weight loss. His physical exam is completely unremarkable. His medications include aspirin, amiodarone, alendronate, metformin, and metoprolol. What is the most likely diagnosis?

   a. Pill-induced esophagitis
   b. Eosinophilic esophagitis from amiodarone
   c. Esophageal candidiasis
   d. Esophageal adenocarcinoma

4. A 40-year-old woman with a presumptive diagnosis of peptic ulcer disease and positive serology for *Helicobacter pylori* has been treated with a proton pump inhibitor and eradication therapy 4 weeks prior. She denies any weight loss, anemia, or occult blood in her stool. Since the initiation of therapy her symptoms, although

somewhat improved, have persisted. You suspect *H. pylori* resistance. What is the next step in management?

a. EGD (esophagogastroduodenoscopy) ± biopsy at this time
b. EGD ± biopsy 8 weeks after the initiation of therapy
c. Repeat *H. pylori* serology
d. *H. pylori* breath test

5. A 35-year-old white man presents with 4 months of weight loss and pruritic rash over his extremities. Physical exam is unremarkable except for a papulovesicular rash. Which of the following is the most appropriate diagnostic test?
   a. Measure antigliadin antibody
   b. Measure immunoglobulin A (IgA) antitissue transglutaminase antibody
   c. EGD and biopsy
   d. Empiric gluten restriction
   e. Skin biopsy
6. A 44-year-old man presents with severe epigastric pain radiating to the back with inability to tolerate any food secondary to pain. A presumptive diagnosis of pancreatitis is made and an abdominal CT (computed tomography) scan shows significant pancreatic inflammation. Vital signs are significant for a temperature 99°F, heart rate 105 beats/min, and blood pressure 100/58 mm Hg. Physical exam is notable for significant epigastric pain on palpation and some guarding but no rebound. Laboratory tests are as follows:

   Hematocrit: 53%
   Leukocyte count: 8000/cu mm
   Platelet count: 300,000/cu mm
   Sodium: 145 mEq/L
   Blood urea nitrogen: 30 mg/dL
   Creatinine: 1.7 mg/dL

   What is the most appropriate next step in management?
   a. Prophylactic imipenem given extent of pancreatic inflammation
   b. Nasogastric decompression
   c. ERCP (endoscopic retrograde cholangiopancreatogram) with sphincterotomy
   d. Fluid resuscitation
7. A 45-year-old woman presents with 8 weeks of loose, watery, large-volume stools. Stool tests:

   Leukocytes: Negative
   Clostridium difficile toxin: Negative
   Ova and parasites: Negative
   pH: 5.2
   Sodium: 80 mEq/L
   Potassium: 30 mEq/L
   Sudan stain: Negative

   What is the possible diagnosis?
   a. Laxative abuse
   b. Irritable bowel syndrome

c. Lactose intolerance
d. Hyperthyroidism

8. A 34-year-old man with ulcerative colitis confined to the rectum since the age of 24 and family history of colon cancer in his mother at the age of 45, which of the following best describes the patient's colon cancer screening strategy?

   a. Annual flexible sigmoidoscopy and fecal occult blood testing at age 35 years
   b. Annual colonoscopy beginning now
   c. Annual colonoscopy starting at age 35 years
   d. Annual flexible sigmoidoscopy with fecal occult blood testing now

9. A 32-year-old obese man presents for a physical examination prior to starting a new job. Routine laboratory test are as follows:
   Alkaline phosphatase: 384 IU/L
   Total bilirubin: 3.2 mg/dL
   AST (aspartate transaminases): 20 U/L
   ALT (alanine aminotransferase): 24 U/L

   What is the most appropriate diagnostic test?

   a. Abdominal ultrasound
   b. ERCP
   c. Hepatitis serology
   d. Bone scan

10. A 20-year-old woman with known ulcerative colitis currently on prednisone 30 mg/day, presents with 1 week of abdominal pain and diarrhea with up to 10 bowel movements. Colonoscopy reveals severe inflammation extending from the rectum to the ileum. The patient is treated with methylprednisolone 26 mg iv BID with no improvement after 4 days. Which of the following is the next step in management?

    a. Intravenous cyclosporine
    b. Increase methylprednisolone dose
    c. Start methotrexate followed by sulfasalazine
    d. Surgery if the patient fails to respond in 5 days

11. A 54-year-old obese woman with end-stage renal disease presents with fever and right upper quadrant pain. Laboratory studies are as follows:
    AST: 200 U/L
    ALT: 250 U/L
    Total bilirubin: 1.2 mg/dL
    Alkaline phosphatase: 340 IU/L
    Leukocyte count: 10,600 cells/mm^3
    Lipase: 300 U/L

    Physical exam is remarkable for right upper quadrant tenderness but without guarding, rigidity, or rebound tenderness. Abdominal ultrasound shows a gallbladder with multiple gallstones but without ductal dilatation and a negative sonographic Murphy sign. Which of the following is the most likely diagnosis?

a. Acute cholecystitis
b. Acute cholangitis
c. Choledocholithiasis
d. Gallstone pancreatitis

12. Which of the following diagnosis is suggested by the following serology?

HBs Ag	Anti-HBs	Anti-HBc antibody	HBeAg	Anti-HBe Antibody	HBV DNA
+	–	IgG	+	–	+

a. Acute hepatitis B
b. Chronic hepatitis B high replication
c. Hepatitis B vaccine
d. Hepatitis B inactive carrier

13. A 45-year-old woman with history of depression presents with a new diagnosis of chronic hepatitis B with HBV DNA 5,000 copies/mL, HBe Ag negative, ALT 25 U/L. What is the next step in the management?

a. No therapy, recheck ALT in 3 months
b. No therapy, recheck ALT in 6 months
c. Initiate treatment with interferon
d. Initiate treatment with lamivudine

14. A 63-year-old man presents with gradual onset right lower quadrant pain and fever. He is treated by his primary care physician with empiric levofloxacin and metronidazole; 4 days later he returns to your office as he is unable to tolerate food secondary to pain. An abdominal CT shows sigmoid diverticulitis and no evidence of an abscess. What is the most appropriate next step in management?

a. Admit to the hospital; continue medical management with intravenous antibiotics
b. Admit to the hospital; continue medical management with a different antibiotic regimen
c. Continue outpatient management with levofloxacin and metronidazole and provide reassurance
d. Surgery

15. A 52-year-old man with a 20-pack-year smoking history presents with epigastric and right upper quadrant pain and 8 lb weight loss for the last 4 months. Abdominal CT shows a 1-cm lesion in the tail of the pancreas. Which of the following diagnostic tests should be performed next?

a. ERCP
b. Magnetic resonance cholangiopancreatogram (MRCP)
c. Endoscopic ultrasound
d. CA 19-9 level

16. A 36-year-old man with ulcerative colitis presents with 6 months of pruritis. His past medical history is otherwise unremarkable. His only medication is sulfasalazine. Physical exam is unremarkable. Laboratory data are as follows:

    White blood cell count: 6,000 cells/mm^3 (polymorphonuclear neutrophils 74%, monocytes 6%, lymphocytes 12%, basophils 4%, eosinophils 4%)
    AST: 30 U/L
    ALT: 30 U/L
    Alkaline phosphatase: 400 IU/L
    Total bilirubin: 2.1 mg/dL
    Direct bilirubin: 1.6 mg/dL

    An abdominal ultrasound is of poor quality secondary to body habitus. What is the most appropriate next step in this patient's management?

    a. Discontinue sulfasalazine
    b. Abdominal MRI
    c. ERCP/MRCP
    d. Hepatitis serology

17. A 45-year-old man presents with dysphagia to solids and liquids for 5 months with regurgitation of swallowed food. He denies any

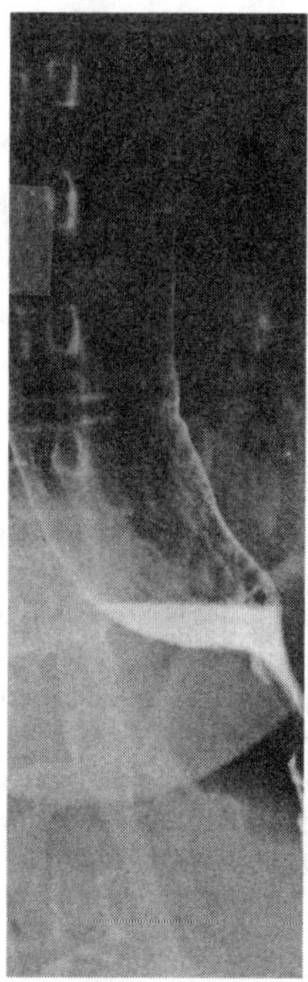

(From Yamada T, Alpers D, Kaplowitz N, et al. *Textbook of gastroenterology*. Vol. 1. 4th ed. Baltimore: Lippincott Williams & Wilkins; 2003:1180, with permission.)

weight loss. A barium swallow image is shown in the figure. What is the most likely diagnosis?

a. Esophageal adenocarcinoma
b. Zenker's diverticulum
c. Esophageal stricture
d. Achalasia cardia

18. A 64-year-old man presents with intermittent mild right upper quadrant discomfort. Physical exam is unremarkable and laboratory studies are as follows:

    Leukocyte count: 6,000 cells/mm^3
    AST: 30 U/L
    ALT: 34 U/L
    Total bilirubin: 1.2 mg/dL

    Abdominal ultrasound reveals gallbladder calcification, no pericholecystic fluid, and no sonographic Murphy sign. Which of the following should be done next?

    a. Start ursodiol
    b. Provide reassurance
    c. Cholecystectomy
    d. ERCP

19. A 65-year-old woman with osteoarthritis, hypertension, and ischemic cardiomyopathy presents to an emergency room with dyspnea and lightheadedness. She is on naprosyn, aspirin, clopidogrel, furosemide, and metoprolol. Laboratory studies are significant for hematocrit of 28. An upper endoscopy reveals a gastric ulcer and serology for *H. pylori* is negative. Which of the following medications should be started?

    a. Start a protein pump inhibitor (PPI) or H2 blocker
    b. Start a PPI
    c. Start sucralfate
    d. Start misoprostol

20. Which of the following statements is true regarding hepatitis?

    a. Chronic hepatitis A results from 10% of acute hepatitis A infections
    b. Chronic hepatitis B results from 10% of acute hepatitis B infections
    c. Chronic hepatitis C results from 10% of acute hepatitis C infections

21. A 46-year-old otherwise healthy woman presents with right upper quadrant and epigastric pain that radiates to the back. She has had mild episodes of intermittent abdominal pain in the past. Abdominal CT shows peripancreatic fat stranding and multiple gallstones. Her temperature is 101°F, heart rate 110 beats/min, and blood pressure 110/60 mm Hg. Laboratory data are as follows:

    Total bilirubin: 2.4 mg/dL
    AST: 30 U/L
    ALT: 25 U/L
    Alkaline phosphatase: 420 IU/L
    Lipase: 500 U/L

Aggressive fluid resuscitation and intravenous antibiotics are started. What is the next step in this patient's management?

a. ERCP with sphincterotomy
b. Nasogastric decompression
c. CT-guided debridement
d. MRCP

22. Which of the following statements pertaining to a cholecystectomy in the prior patient is true?

a. Cholecystectomy should be performed prior to discharge
b. Cholecystectomy is unnecessary if an ERCP with sphincterotomy has been performed
c. Cholecystectomy is necessary if the patient fails a course of ursodeoxycholeic acid
d. An emergent cholecystectomy should be performed

23. A 59-year-old woman with left-sided back pain has evidence of a renal calculus and a gallstone on abdominal CT scan (without contrast). She denies any abdominal pain, nausea, vomiting, or fever. Ultrasound confirms the presence of gallstones but there is no cholecystic fluid or thickening of the gallbladder wall. What is the next step in the patient's management with regard to the gallstone?

a. Lithotripsy for both the renal calculus and the gallstone
b. Ursodeoxycholeic acid for dissolution of the gallstone
c. Referral for laparoscopic cholecystectomy
d. Reassurance

24. A 72-year-old man with coronary artery disease, hypertension, dyslipidemia, and diabetes mellitus presents to an emergency room with severe periumbilical pain without radiation. He reports having similar episodes in the past that are brought on with meals and has lost 7 lb in the last 5 months. A trial of proton pump inhibitors prescribed by his primary care physician has provided no relief. On palpation his abdomen is minimally tender to palpation, no organomegaly and normal bowel sounds, on rectal exam he is guiaic negative. What is the next step in management?

a. Initiation of a heparin drip
b. Right upper quadrant and renal ultrasound
c. Trial of H2 blockers, viscous lidocaine, and kaopectate for immediate relief
d. Abdominal CT with angiography

25. A 58-year-old man presents to the emergency room with 72 hours of left lower quadrant abdominal pain and has been unable to tolerate food secondary to the pain. An abdominal CT scan performed 2 days prior showed evidence of diverticulitis, and oral antibiotic treatment with levofloxacin and metronidazole was initiated. Repeat abdominal CT shows persistent diverticulitis with no evidence of fluid collection and is essentially unchanged. He is hospitalized for intravenous antibiotics and 72 hours later is afebrile with improvement in

abdominal pain and can tolerate solid food. Which of the following is the most appropriate next step in management?

a. Discharge the patient from the hospital, continue antibiotics for total of 10 days, and arrange an outpatient colonoscopy in 2 months
b. Continue antibiotics for total of 7 days and arrange an inpatient colonoscopy prior to discharge
c. Continue antibiotics for total of 10 days and arrange an inpatient flexible sigmoidoscopy prior to discharge
d. Discharge the patient; continue oral antibiotics for a total of 14 days, and follow-up abdominal CT scan 1 week after discharge

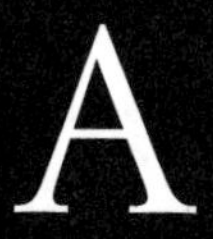

Appendix A

Answers

1. **a**	10. **b**	19. **b**
2. **d**	11. **b**	20. **b**
3. **d**	12. **b**	21. **a**
4. **d**	13. **b**	22. **a**
5. **b**	14. **a**	23. **d**
6. **d**	15. **c**	24. **d**
7. **c**	16. **c**	25. **a**
8. **c**	17. **d**	
9. **a**	18. **c**	

1. **a.** GERD is a clinical diagnosis. It is appropriate to begin empiric treatment with acid suppression therapy. In patients who do not respond to acid suppression and in whom the diagnosis is uncertain, 24-h pH probe or barium swallow is indicated. Patients with longstanding reflux 8 to 10 years it has been recommended to perform an EGD for surveillance for Barrett's esophagus. In patients who do not wish to continue lifelong acid suppression and in whom there is confirmed reflux are candidates for antireflux surgery.
2. **d.** Patients with suspected peptic ulcer disease > 45 years of age, anemia, weight loss, anorexia, or positive fecal occult blood should have an upper endoscopy and biopsy to rule out gastric cancer. For patients without the above symptoms, PPI therapy can be initiated and patients tested and treated for *H. pylori* if they are found to have positive serology. Discontinuation of aspirin therapy in patients with known coronary artery disease may be needed depending on EGD findings but should not be the first step. The prescription of misoprostol is indicated only in patients with previous ulcers induced by nonsteroidal anti-inflammatory drugs (NSAIDs), and is not the most appropriate step at this time.
3. **d.** Although pill-induced esophagitis is associated with bisphosphonates such as alendronate, it is not associated with the weight loss. In a patient with no underlying immunocompromised state it would be unusual to have esophageal candidiasis without evidence of oral thrush. Eosinophilic esophagitis is rare and should be suspected when patients have a lack of response to acid suppression in addition to mucosal and peripheral eosinophilia and elevated IgE levels.

Given the dysphagia to solids, significant weight loss, and history of longstanding reflux, esophageal adenocarcinoma is the most likely diagnosis.

4. **d.** Patients less than 45 years of age with suspected peptic ulcer disease without alarm symptoms (weight loss, anorexia, anemia, occult blood in stool) should have noninvasive tests for *H. pylori* (serology or breath test) followed by eradication therapy if positive. An EGD in recommended if patients fail to respond in 8 weeks and confirmation of *H. pylori* should be done with a biopsy at the time of the EGD. *Helicobacter pylori* serology is used only to make an initial diagnosis of infection; follow-up to confirm eradication is with a breath test as serology remains positive.
5. **b.** Tissue transglutaminase antibody is sensitive and specific for celiac sprue. IgA and IgG antigliadin antibody tests have lower diagnostic accuracy with frequent false-positive results and are not recommended for initial diagnostic evaluation or screening. An EGD and biopsy are recommended when serology for sprue is positive. If both serology and biopsy confirm the diagnosis of celiac sprue, patients should be instructed to avoid gluten. The clinical presentation suggests the diagnosis of celiac sprue, and a skin biopsy is not necessary to establish the diagnosis.
6. **d.** The patient's laboratory data suggest that there is significant hemoconcentration secondary to third spacing of fluid. Prior studies have demonstrated that fluid resuscitation has not been shown to prevent pancreatic necrosis, but all patients with persistent hemoconcentration at 24 hours develop necrotizing pancreatitis. Aggressive intravenous hydration to ensure hematocrit $< 44\%$ is therefore the first step in management. Prophylactic imipenem has been shown to decrease the incidence of pancreatic sepsis in patients with necrotizing pancreatitis. The abdominal CT scan does not show evidence of pancreatic necrosis and is not indicated at this time. ERCP with sphincterotomy performed within 24 hours of admission has been shown to decrease the incidence of biliary sepsis in patients with gallstone pancreatitis. Nasogastric tube decompression is not needed in all cases of pancreatitis but should be used in those patients with persistent emesis and ileus.
7. **c.** Osmotic Gap $= 290 - 2(\text{Na} + \text{K}) = 290 - 2(110) = 70$; Gap > 50 mOsm suggests osmotic diarrhea and a pH < 5.5 suggests carbohydrate malabsorption. Laxative abuse, hyperparathyroidism, and irritable bowel syndrome are associated with a normal osmotic gap.
8. **c.** This patient has two risk factors for colon cancer: family history of colon cancer and a longstanding history of ulcerative colitis. Given the early age at cancer diagnosis in a first-degree relative, the patient should undergo colon cancer screening 10 years prior to that diagnosis, i.e., at age 35 years. His mother should also be genetically tested for hereditary nonpolyposis colorectal cancer given the early

age of onset of colon cancer (<50 years). Recommended colon cancer screening in patients with longstanding ulcerative colitis consists of colonoscopy every 1 to 2 years after 8 years in patients with pancolitis and after 15 years in patients with left-sided colitis. Flexible sigmoidoscopy carries the risk of missing right-sided colon cancer, therefore making colonoscopy the recommended screening test.

9. **a.** Elevation in AST, ALT, and alkaline phosphatase suggests a hepatic cause of elevated alkaline phosphatase. Elevations in alkaline phosphatase that are greater than threefold merit imaging of the biliary tree with an abdominal ultrasound followed by an ERCP if ductal dilatation is seen on ultrasound. A bone scan would be indicated if there were an elevation in alkaline phosphatase with normal liver function tests, suggesting a bone source.

10. **b.** Oral prednisone or prednisolone is used for induction of remission in moderately severe ulcerative colitis or Crohn's disease. Intravenous administration is indicated in patients with severe ulcerative colitis. Patients who fail to respond to steroids should be treated with cyclosporine. Failure to respond after 7 to 10 days of cyclosporine therapy, perforation, toxic megacolon, hemorrhage and systemic complications, dysplasia/cancer are indications for surgery. There is no indication for the use of methotrexate in patients with ulcerative colitis.

11. **b.** The presence of fever, an elevated white count, and right upper quadrant pain suggests the presence of an infection in the gallbladder/biliary tree. Neither choledocholithiasis (presence of stones in the biliary tree) or gallstone pancreatitis is associated with a leukocytosis and fever. Furthermore, in patients with end-stage renal disease there must be a threefold elevation in lipase to make a diagnosis of pancreatitis. In patients with bile duct obstruction secondary to a gallstones, an elevated AST and ALT with alkaline phosphatase may be seen even before elevations in bilirubin. This patient certainly has choledocholithiasis with an infection of the biliary tree, making the most likely diagnosis acute cholangitis.

12. **b.** Patients with acute hepatitis B are positive for anti-HBc IgM antibody. The presence of anti-HBc IgG antibody suggests chronic hepatitis. Presence of HBeAg and absence of HBe antibody suggests active viral replication. Following immunization with hepatitis B patients are anti-HBs antibody positive and HBsAg, HBeAg, and Anti-HBc antibody are negative.

13. **b.** Inactive chronic hepatitis B carriers (HBs Ag^+, HBe Ag^- and normal ALT) can be followed with ALT every 6 months, if ALT > 2 times normal, HBV DNA levels should be checked. If at that time the patient is found to have elevated HBV DNA (>10^5 copies/mL), treatment can be initiated. Interferon is contraindicated in patients with depression and either lamivudine or adefovir can be used to treat these patients.

14. **a.** The patient should be admitted to the hospital for intravenous antibiotics as he is unable to tolerate oral medications. Given that the patient has only been on the current antibiotic regimen for 4 days, it should be continued as there is no evidence of antibiotic failure at this time. There is no evidence of an abscess on the abdominal CT scan and therefore no indication for surgery at this time.

15. **c.** Endoscopic ultrasound is the test of choice for a pancreatic lesion in the tail of the pancreas and allows for a biopsy to be taken. MRCP and ERCP are both of diagnostic utility in cases where a pancreatic cancer is suspected and CT is negative for a mass but still suspected or pancreatic ductal strictures are present. CA 19-9 is a tumor marker and is not a diagnostic test for pancreatic cancer. It has a sensitivity that approaches 80% but may be elevated in the absence of pancreatic cancer. It is therefore used to follow patients after resection of pancreatic cancer.

16. **c.** This patient with ulcerative colitis likely has sclerosing cholangitis. There is no evidence of peripheral eosinophilia or skin rash and therefore discontinuing sulfasalazine that is indicated for maintenance therapy of ulcerative colitis is not necessary. Given the elevated alkaline phosphatase and cholestatic picture, further imaging of the biliary tree is indicated with an ERCP/MRCP that can demonstrate both intrahepatic and extrahepatic ductal dilatation. Hepatitis serologies would be indicated if the patient had elevated transaminases.

17. **d.** The barium swallow in the radiograph shows esophageal dilatation with an air fluid level and a smoothly tapering esophagus, which is characteristic of achalasia. By the clinical presentation it is possible to narrow the differential as well. Dysphagia to solids and liquids suggests the presence of a motility disorder. Esophageal adenocarcinoma and strictures produce gradually progressive dysphagia to solids that then progress to dysphagia to liquids. Zenker's diverticulum produces intermittent dysphagia.

18. **c.** This patient has gallbladder calcification (porcelain gallbladder), which is a premalignant condition and therefore warrants a cholecystectomy. Ursodeoxycholeic acid is used to treat patients with gallstones who are not surgical candidates. There is no evidence for a biliary obstruction, making an ERCP unnecessary.

19. **b.** Proton pump inhibitor is superior to H2 blockers, sucralfate, and misoprostol in NSAID-induced ulcer healing.

20. **b.** Hepatitis A is not associated with a chronic phase. Of acute infections in adults, 5% to 10% result in a chronic hepatitis B; 80% to 100% of patients with acute hepatitis C develop chronic hepatitis C.

21. **a.** This patient has pancreatitis secondary to gallstones and possibly cholangitis from biliary obstruction. Although there is no evidence of ductal dilatation, this may not be seen in the early stages and there may be obstruction from sludge in the biliary tree that can be

cleared with an ERCP. An MRCP would not provide any therapeutic intervention. CT-guided debridement would be necessary if there were infected pancreatic tissue, which is not seen in the abdominal CT. Nasogastric decompression is indicated in patients with severe pancreatitis with evidence of ileus.

22. **a.** Given the presence of multiple gallstones within the gallbladder, even with a sphincterotomy the patient is at risk for a recurrent episode of gallstone pancreatitis. A cholecystectomy is not emergent but should therefore be performed at prior to discharge. Patients with symptomatic gallstones who are not operative candidates may be treated with ursodeoxycholeic acid ± ERCP with sphincterotomy.

23. **d.** This patient is asymptomatic, and therefore treatment of cholelithiasis is not indicated. Patients with symptomatic cholelithiasis or complications, who are surgical candidates, should undergo cholecystectomy. Patients with symptomatic cholelithiasis, who are not operative candidates, may be treated with ursodeoxycholeic acid ± ERCP with sphincterotomy.

24. **d.** The patient has known vascular disease and symptoms are consistent with mesenteric ischemia. Abdominal pain with severe pain out of proportion to the physical exam. Small bowel ischemia pain is usually periumbilical. Pain is usually sudden in onset with embolic occlusion but may be gradual with thrombosis or vasospasm. Abdominal CT with intravenous contrast or angiography is useful in making a diagnosis. Angiography is both diagnostic and therapeutic, as are embolectomy, thrombolysis, thrombectomy, the use of vasodilators in patients with NOMI (nonocclusive mesenteric ischemia), or provides important information for an arterial bypass.

25. **a.** Once the patient is tolerating oral medication and is afebrile, it is appropriate to discharge him from the hospital and continue antibiotics for a total of 7 to 10 days. Colonoscopy or flexible sigmoidoscopy is not performed in patients with acute diverticulitis due to the risk of perforation. However, an outpatient colonoscopy in 2 months is warranted to exclude the presence of a malignancy in the area that was not seen on CT scan.

Appendix

B Opportunities in Gastroenterology

Gastroenterology is a subspecialty of internal medicine. In 2006, 134 programs committed 283 positions in the GI match. Gastroenterology fellowship is one of the most competitive fellowships in the country. A comprehensive list of programs can be found online at www.nrmp.org or www.ama-assn.org. There are four possible fellowship tracks within gastroenterology: Clinical, Clinical Investigator, Basic Science Research, and Research.

Fellowship in gastroenterology involves an average of 3 years of training after the completion of 3 years of internal medicine residency. Of the 3 years, 18 months are designated clinical rotations consisting of inpatient, consultative gastrointestinal/hepatology service and outpatient gastroenterology and hepatology. The remainder of the 3 years depends on the fellowship program and the individual track.

The gastroenterology fellowship match has been reinstituted in 2005–2006 and is subject to change. For the most recent information on the gastroenterology fellowship match, visit http://www.gastro.org.

The approximate time line for the match is as follows:

- Fall–Winter: Residents apply to fellowship programs by manually submitting applications to individual fellowship programs. Most deadlines are December 15 to January 1.
- January: National Residency Matching Program online registration for programs and applicants begins.
- January–April: Fellowship interviews for applicants.
- April: Rank order list opens.
- June: Rank order list certification for applicants and programs.
- End of June: Match Day.

How to Obtain a Gastroenterology Fellowship Position

Fellowship program directors are looking for applicants with strong academic credentials from premiere residency programs. In addition, previous gastroenterology clinical and research experience, as well as strong letters of support are important. The personal statement in the gastroenterology application is akin to a statement of purpose and should serve to highlight the applicant's anticipated goals as a future gastroenterologist.

Electives in gastroenterology during the first 2 years of residency are a valuable way of confirming your interest, demonstrating your commitment to the field, and obtaining letters of recommendation from gastroenterologists.

Prior research experience, although not essential, will certainly help to bolster your fellowship application. A significant number of applicants often have research experience prior to medical school. Finding a research project during the first 2 years of residency and developing a broad area of interest in gastroenterology (liver or luminal pathology; basic or clinical research) could serve to give you an edge over other applicants. Expressing an area of interest will help fellowship directors match you with faculty at their institutions at an interview.

Interviews at many gastroenterology programs consist of five to seven interviews approximately 30 minutes each. Fellowship program directors use the interviews to gauge a candidate's interest in gastroenterology, current research, future interests, and career goals. The interview day also represents an excellent opportunity to speak with fellows who can give you valuable insight into the program.

Good Luck!

Appendix

C Commonly Prescribed Medications and Dosage

This appendix lists some commonly prescribed medications in gastroenterology. This list is by no means comprehensive or exhaustive. Indications and contraindications must be carefully considered before prescribing any of the following medications. The doses listed below are an approximation and, as medicine is an ever-changing field, doses of all medications listed below must be verified with the manufacturer's package insert. Patient age, hepatic, renal impairment, interaction with other medications, side effects, and the clinical condition must be taken into account and dose adjustments made accordingly before they are prescribed. Patients must be monitored by a physician while on treatment.

Histamine-2 Receptor Blockers (H2 Blockers)

- Ranitidine
  - Prevention of heartburn (over-the-counter, OTC) 75 mg 30–60 min before a meal, maximum 150 mg in 24 h, not to be used for more than 14 days
  - Peptic ulcers 150 mg PO TID or 300 mg PO q day, maintenance 150 mg QHS
  - Erosive esophagitis: 150 mg QID, maintenance 150 mg BID

Proton Pump Inhibitors

- Omeprazole
  - Peptic ulcer disease: 20–40 mg q day for 4–8 weeks
  - Gastroesophageal reflux disease: 20 mg q day for 4 weeks
  - Erosive esophagitis: 20 mg q day for 4–8 weeks
- Esomeprazole
  - Peptic ulcer disease: 40 mg q day in combination with eradication of *Helicobacter pylori*
  - Gastroesophageal reflux disease: 20 mg q day for 4 weeks
  - Erosive esophagitis: 20–40 mg q day or BID for 4–8 weeks

Helicobacter pylori **Infection**

- Lansoprazole 30 mg, amoxicillin 1 g, and clarithromycin 500 mg taken together twice daily for 10 or 14 days
- Bismuth subsalicylate 524.8-mg tablet, metronidazole 250-mg tablet, and tetracycline 500-mg capsule plus an H2 antagonist four times/day at meals and bedtime for 14 days

Esophageal Variceal Bleeding

- Octreotide: Intravenous bolus: 25–50 μg followed by continuous infusion 25–50 μg/h

Diarrhea

- Antimotility agents
  - Loperamide: Acute diarrhea. Initial: 4 mg, followed by 2 mg after each loose stool, up to 16 mg/day
  - Diphenoxylate: Oral: 5 mg PO TID

Constipation

- Bulk laxative
  - Methylcellulose: 19 g powder in 8 oz water q day-TID
- Stool softener
  - Docusate: 50–500 mg/day in one to four divided doses
- Osmotic laxative
  - Lactulose for constipation: 15–30 mL BID
  - Lactulose for hepatic encephalopathy: 30–45 mL q 1–2 hours to induce rapid laxation and then decreased to 30 mL QID
- Stimulant laxative
  - Senna: 15 mg q day–QID

Gastroparesis

- Metoclopramide: 10 mg QID (30 min before each meal and at bedtime) for 2–8 weeks

Irritable Bowel Syndrome

- Tegaserod: For treatment of constipation-predominant irritable bowel syndrome in women
  - 6 mg PO BID before meals, for 4–6 weeks

Inflammatory Bowel Disease

5-ASA Drugs

- Mesalamine for ileitis and colitis in inflammatory bowel disease
  - Initial treatment: 800 mg PO TID for 6 weeks
  - Maintenance: 1.6 g/day in divided doses
  - Rectal suppositories for proctitis: 500 mg suppository BID–TID
- Sulfasalazine for colitis in inflammatory bowel disease
  - Initial: 1 g PO TID–QID
  - Maintenance: 2 g/day in divided doses

Antibiotics in Crohn's Disease

- Metronidazole in ileocolitis and colitis in Crohn's disease, Oral: 10–20 mg/kg/day in divided doses

Corticosteroids

- Prednisone in patients with severe Crohn's disease. Oral: 40–60 mg/day and should then be tapered. Failure to respond to oral prednisone should be treated with intravenous methylprednisolone 10–40 mg q 4–6 hours for 48 h

Immunomodulators

- Azathioprine: Oral, 2.5 mg/kg per day (maximum)
- 6-Mercaptopurine: Oral, 50 mg/day–2 mg/kg/day (maximum)
- Infliximab in Crohn's disease
  - Initial: 5 mg/kg at 0, 2, and 6 weeks, followed by 5 mg/kg every 8 weeks; dose may be increased to 10 mg/kg in patients who respond but then lose their response.

Suggested Reading

Esophagus

Fass R, Fennerty MB, et al. Nonerosive reflux disease—current concepts and dilemmas. *Am J Gastroenterol* 2001;96(2):303–314.

Penagini RS, Carmagnola, et al. Review article: gastro-oesophageal reflux disease—pathophysiological issues of clinical relevance. *Aliment Pharmacol Ther* 2002;16(Suppl. 4):65–71.

Richter JE. Oesophageal motility disorders. *Lancet* 2001;358(9284): 823–828.

Spechler SJ. Intestinal metaplasia at the gastroesophageal junction. *Gastroenterology* 2004;126(2):567–575.

Vaezi MF, Richter JE. Diagnosis and management of achalasia. American College of Gastroenterology Practice Parameter Committee. *Am J Gastroenterol* 1999;94(12):3406–3412.

Gastroenterology Imaging

Adamek HE, Breer H, et al. Magnetic resonance cholangiopancreatography. The fine art of bilio-pancreatic imaging. *Pancreatology* 2002; 2(6):499–502.

Byrne MF, Jowell PS. Gastrointestinal imaging: endoscopic ultrasound. *Gastroenterology* 2002;122(6):1631–1648.

Liver and Gall Bladder

Angulo, P. Nonalcoholic fatty liver disease. *N Engl J Med* 2002;346(16): 1221–1231.

Arroyo V, Guevara M, et al. Hepatorenal syndrome in cirrhosis: pathogenesis and treatment. *Gastroenterology* 2002;122(6):1658–1676.

Befeler AS, Di Bisceglie AM. Hepatocellular carcinoma: diagnosis and treatment. *Gastroenterology* 2002;122(6):1609–1619.

Bruno R, Sacchi P, et al. HCV chronic hepatitis in patients with HIV: clinical management issues. *Am J Gastroenterol* 2002; 97(7):1598–1606.

Gores JJ. Cholangiocarcinoma: current concepts and insights. *Hepatology* 2003;37(5):961–969.

Grace ND. Diagnosis and treatment of gastrointestinal bleeding secondary to portal hypertension. American College of Gastroenterology Practice Parameters Committee.[see comment]. *Am J Gastroenterol* 1997;92(7):1081–1091.

Jensen DM. Endoscopic screening for varices in cirrhosis: findings, implications, and outcomes. *Gastroenterology.* 2002;122(6):1620–1630.

Maher JJ. Treatment of alcoholic hepatitis. *J Gastroenterol Hepatol* 2002;17(4):448–455.

Moore KP, Wong F, et al. The management of ascites in cirrhosis: report on the consensus conference of the International Ascites Club. *Hepatology* 2003;38(1):258–266.

Runyon BA. Albumin infusion for spontaneous bacterial peritonitis. *Lancet* 1999;354(9193):1838–1839.

Runyon BA. Management of adult patients with ascites caused by cirrhosis. *Hepatology* 1998;27(1):264–272.

Sandhu BS, Sanyal AJ. Pregnancy and liver disease. *Gastroenterol Clin North Am* 2003;32(1):407–436, ix.

Sanyal AJ. American Gastroenterological AGA technical review on nonalcoholic fatty liver disease. *Gastroenterology* 2002;123(5):1705–1725.

Sobhonslidsuk A, Reddy KR. Portal vein thrombosis: a concise review. *Am J Gastroenterol* 2002;97(3):535–541.

Trowbridge RL, Rutkowski NK, et al. Does this patient have acute cholecystitis? *JAMA* 2003;289(1):80–86.

Zeuzem S, Heathcote E, Shiffman M, et al. Twelve weeks of follow-up is sufficient for the determination of sustained virologic response in patients treated with interferon á for chronic hepatitis C. *J Hepatol* 2003;39(1):106–111.

Pancreas

Banks PA. Practice guidelines in acute pancreatitis. *Am J Gastroenterol* 1997;92(3):377–386.

Brown A, Baillargeon J, Hughes MD, et al. Can Fluid Resuscitation Prevent Pancreatic Necrosis in Severe Acute Pancreatitis? *Pancreatol* 2002;2: 104–107.

DiMagno EP, Reber HA, et al. AGA technical review on the epidemiology, diagnosis, and treatment of pancreatic ductal adenocarcinoma. American Gastroenterological Association. *Gastroenterology* 1999; 117(6):1464–1484.

Etemad B, Whitcomb DC. Chronic pancreatitis: diagnosis, classification, and new genetic developments. *Gastroenterology* 2001;120(3):682–707.

Fan S, Lai E, Mok F, et al. Early Treatment of Acute Biliary Pancreatitis by Endoscopic Papillotomy. *N Engl J Med* 1993;328:228–232.

Fogel EL, Sherman S. Acute biliary pancreatitis: when should the endoscopist intervene? *Gastroenterology* 2003;125(1):229–235.

Lankisch PG. Natural course of chronic pancreatitis. *Pancreatology* 2001;1(1):3–14.

Levy MJ, Geenen JE. Idiopathic acute recurrent pancreatitis. A*m J Gastroenterol* 2001;96(9):2540–2555.

Somogyi L, Martin SP, et al. Recurrent acute pancreatitis: an algorithmic approach to identification and elimination of inciting factors. *Gastroenterology* 2001;120(3):708–717.

Werner J, Hartwig W, et al. Useful markers for predicting severity and monitoring progression of acute pancreatitis. *Pancreatology* 2003;3(2): 115–127.

Small and Large Intestine

Baron JA, Beach M, Mandel JS, et al. Calcium Supplements for the Prevention of Colorectal Adenomas. *N Engl J Med* 1999;340:101–107.

Farrell RJ, Kelly CP. Celiac sprue. *N Engl J Med* 2002;346(3):180–188.

Friedman S, Regueiro MD. Pregnancy and nursing in inflammatory bowel disease. *Gastroenterol Clin North Am* 2002;31(1):265–273.

Friedman S, Rubin PH, et al. Screening and surveillance colonoscopy in chronic Crohn's colitis. *Gastroenterology* 2001;120(4):820–826.

Laine L, Hanauer SB. Considerations in the management of steroid-dependent Crohn's disease. *Gastroenterology* 2003;125(3):906–910.

Modlin IM, Sandor A. An analysis of 8305 cases of carcinoid tumors. *Cancer* 1997;79(4):813–829.

Podolsky DK. Medical progress: inflammatory bowel disease. *N Engl J Med* 2002;(347):417–429.

Ruemmele FM, Targan SR, Levy G, et al. Diagnostic accuracy of serological assays in pediatric inflammatory bowel disease. *Gastroenterology* 1998;115(4):822–829.

Sandborn WJ, Hanauer SB. Infliximab in the treatment of Crohn's disease: a user's guide for clinicians. *Am J Gastroenterol* 2002;97(12): 2962–2972.

Stomach and Duodenum

Quan C, Talley NJ. Management of peptic ulcer disease not related to *Helicobacter pylori* or NSAIDs. *Am J Gastroenterol* 2002;97(12): 2950–2961.

Rubin CE. Are there three types of *Helicobacter pylori* gastritis? *Gastroenterology* 1997;112(6):2108–2110.

Suerbaum S, Michetti P. *Helicobacter pylori* infection. *N Engl J Med* 2002;347(15):1175–1186.

Talley NJ, Silverstein MD, et al. AGA technical review: evaluation of dyspepsia. American Gastroenterological Association. *Gastroenterology* 1998;114(3):582–595.

Witting MD, Magder L, Heins AE, et al. ED predictors of upper gastrointestinal tract bleeding in patients without hematemesis. *Am J Emerg Med* 2006;24(3):259–396.

Index

Page numbers followed by *f* or *t* refer to illustrations or tables, respectively.